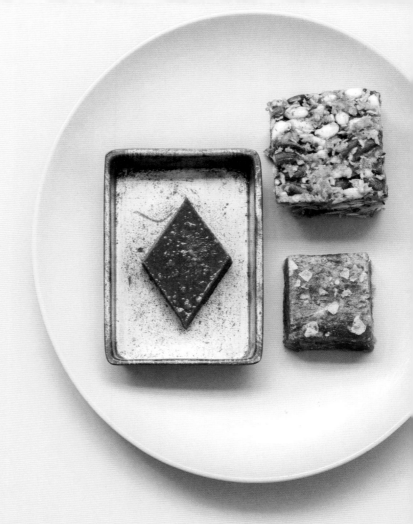

SUPERFOOD
ENERGY BALLS & BITES

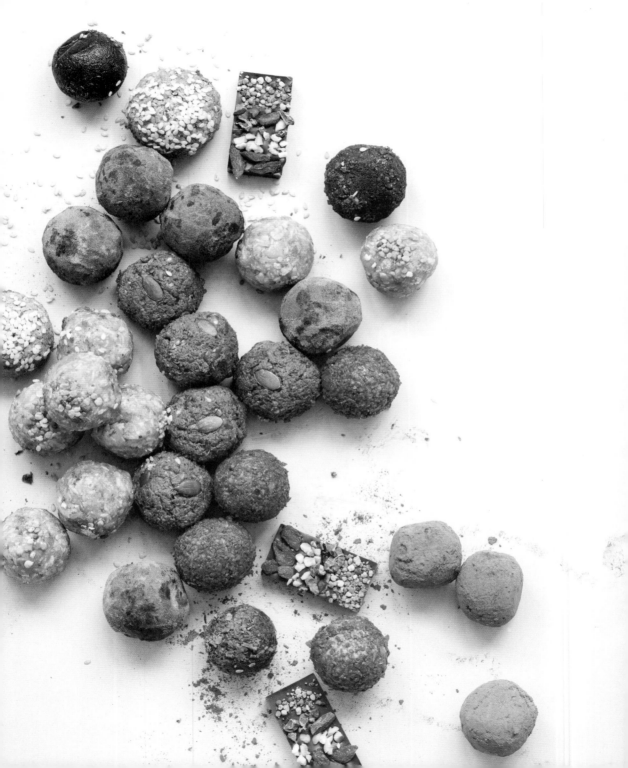

SUPERFOOD
ENERGY BALLS & BITES

Nutrient-rich, healthful & wholesome snacks

Nicola Graimes

Photography by Clare Winfield

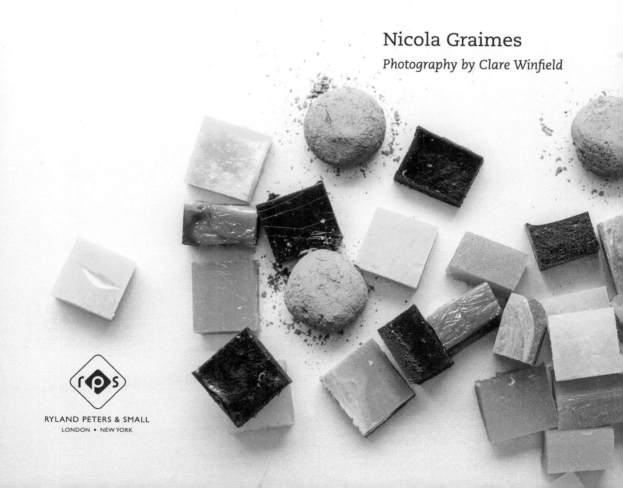

RYLAND PETERS & SMALL
LONDON • NEW YORK

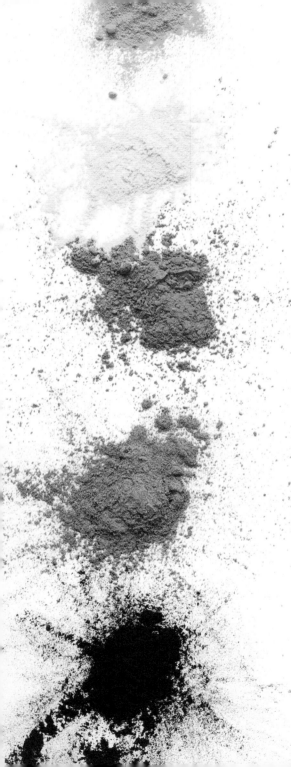

Dedication
To Silvio, Ella & Joel, with love

Senior designer Megan Smith
Editors Miriam Catley and Kate Reeves-Brown
Production manager Gordana Simakovic
Art director Leslie Harrington
Editorial director Julia Charles
Publisher Cindy Richards

Food stylists Maud Eden and Ellie Mulligan
Prop stylist Alexander Breeze
Indexer Vanessa Bird

First published in 2018 by
Ryland Peters & Small
20–21 Jockey's Fields, London WC1R 4BW
and 341 E 116th St, New York NY 10029

www.rylandpeters.com

10 9 8 7 6 5 4 3 2 1

Text copyright © Nicola Graimes 2018
Design and photographs copyright
© Ryland Peters & Small 2018

ISBN: 978-1-84975-929-8

Printed in China

A CIP record for this book is available from the British
Library. US Library of Congress Cataloging-in-Publication
Data has been applied for.

Notes
• Both Metric and Imperial measurements are included in
these recipes for your convenience, however it is advisable
to work with one set of measurements only.
• All spoon measurements are level unless otherwise
specified. A teaspoon is 5 ml, a tablespoon is 15 ml.
• When a recipe calls for the grated zest of citrus fruit, buy
unwaxed fruit and wash well before using.
• Always consult your health advisor or doctor if you have
any concerns about your health or nutrition. Neither the
author nor the publisher can be held responsible for any
claims arising out of the information given in this book.

CONTENTS

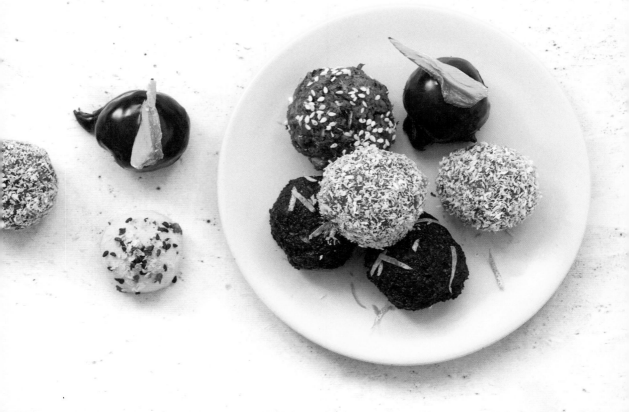

INTRODUCTION

Snacks aren't all bad and the 'right' snack can play a valuable part in a healthy, nutritionally balanced diet. When energy levels are at a low point, you're feeling peckish or need a post-workout boost, a nutrient-rich snack eaten midway between breakfast and lunch and/or between lunch and dinner can give you a much-needed lift.

The list of health benefits is impressive: sustained amounts of energy; even mood; enhanced concentration and focus; stable blood-sugar levels and metabolism; and optimum body functioning. What's more, sensible snacking can help you resist the urge to overeat at mealtimes so can assist in weight control.

Add a 'superfood' to your healthy snack and you have a winning combination. Although 'superfood' may have become a buzzword in recent times, certain foods are undeniably blessed in that they provide superior nutritional value for the amount of calories they contain. This means they can give your snacks a significant health boost, ranging from vitamins, minerals and antioxidants to good fats, good-quality protein, complex carbs and fibre.

More specifically, protein is essential for muscle repair and body maintenance and also increases the production of neurotransmitters that regulate concentration and alertness.

Complex carbs help to lift mood by boosting serotonin levels, provide fibre and are a stable source of energy. While plant foods rich in omega-3 fatty acids, such as flaxseeds (linseeds), walnuts and chia seeds, are welcome additions, benefitting both the heart and brain, and are also good for joint problems and low mood.

Raw and cooked, sweet and savoury, these delicious recipes for energy balls, bars and bites are all easy to make, nutrient-rich and prepared with wholesome ingredients.

These convenient, portable snacks have been created to provide a boost of energy at much-needed times of the day and to suit different dietary requirements. There are recipes suited to pre- and post-workouts, ideas for morning boosters, lunchboxes and after-school snacks, and creations to lift flagging energy levels during an afternoon lull – there is even a collection of delicious bite-sized treats, all with a healthy dose of superfoods. Enjoy!

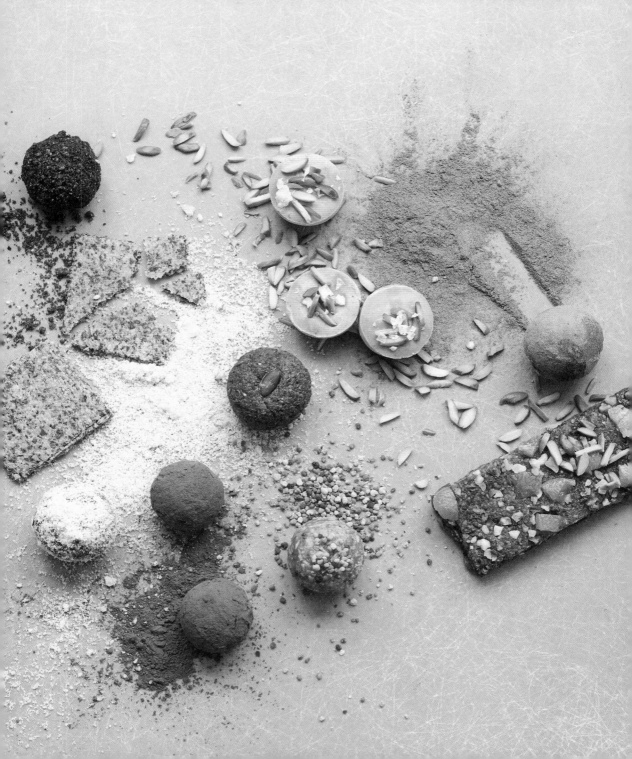

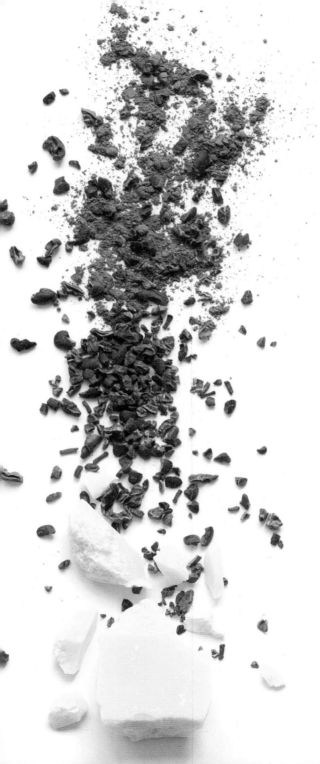

A-Z OF SUPERFOODS

This collection of potent, nutrient-rich superfoods features in the following snack bars, balls and bites, and they have been specifically chosen for their energizing, rejuvenating and uplifting properties. The list isn't exhaustive, as 'new' superfoods often come to our attention, plus you could argue that fruit, vegetables, nuts and seeds should also form part of the list. Yet what they all share is the ability to enhance health, energy levels and well-being, if eaten on a regular basis.

ACAI BERRY

Deep purple in colour with a slightly fruity chocolaty flavour, this Amazonian fruit contains a high concentration of antioxidants – double that of blueberries – meaning it has the ability to neutralize free radicals in the body. Free radicals damage glands and cells making us more prone to disease and ageing. Alongside an impressive vitamin C content, acai berries are a good source of essential fatty acids, fibre and protein, which help to boost energy levels, as well as promote muscle performance, endurance and strength – a perfect combination pre-workout or as a pick-me-up if energy levels are low.

AVOCADO

There was a time when the avocado fell out of favour, mainly due to its high fat content, but how times change. The fruit is now firmly part of the superfood gang thanks to its heart-friendly monounsaturated fat content, along with vitamins C, E and K, magnesium, potassium, iron, copper and folate. Rich and creamy in flavour and consistency, avocados can help with appetite control, since their fat content means they keep us full for longer and provide welcome amounts of energy.

BAOBAB

A relative superfood newcomer outside its country of origin, in Africa the fruit from the baobab tree is rich in ancient myth and legend. Packed with vitamin C – reputedly six times as much as found in an orange – it is also a good source of potassium, iron and magnesium. Baobab is said to help boost energy levels and support the immune system, and has prebiotic qualities that increase levels of good bacteria in the gut. It has a slightly sharp, zingy, citrus flavour.

BEE POLLEN

The diminutive size of these golden 'grains' belies their impressive nutrient content – bee pollen is said to include nearly all the nutrients required by man. Particularly rich in protein – it contains around 40 per cent – bee pollen also provides valuable amounts of vitamins, minerals, antioxidants and fatty acids. Furthermore, it supports the immune system, helps energy production and aids digestion, respiration and circulation. When used in foods, it provides a lovely, intense honey taste and natural sweetness. Word of warning, if you suffer from a pollen allergy, do be mindful when you first try it, as it may cause a similar allergic reaction.

BUCKWHEAT (FLAKES)

Despite its name, buckwheat is not related to wheat and is actually a seed. Gluten-free, buckwheat comes in many forms, but the flakes are used in this book to add high-quality protein, fibre, B vitamins, magnesium and manganese to both sweet and savoury bars and balls.

CACAO (RAW POWDER AND NIBS)

Raw cacao powder may look the same as regular cocoa, but nutritionally they are worlds apart. Made by cold-pressing unroasted cocoa beans, raw cacao retains higher levels of nutrients, especially antioxidants, than regular beans, which are processed at a higher temperature. Raw cacao is one of the richest sources of magnesium, the mineral essential for strong muscles, bones and teeth, while its theobromine (a natural stimulant) content may help to elevate mood and energy levels. Both the powder and nibs (broken up pieces of raw cacao bean) are used in the recipes with the latter adding a pleasant crunch.

CACAO BUTTER (PURE OR RAW)

This creamy-coloured, solid vegetable fat comes from the cocoa bean and unsurprisingly has a taste and aroma of chocolate. Raw or pure cacao butter is preferential since it hasn't been heated to a high temperature and subsequently retains more of its healthy fats and high antioxidant content, particularly immune-boosting polyphenols and flavonoids. You can buy it in chunks or buttons, ready for blending or melting, and it's particularly good in energy balls and bars since it sets when cool, helping to hold everything together. It's also a great skin moisturiser!

CHIA SEEDS

A wonder food... the nutritional value of this tiny seed is impressive. It is one of the richest plant sources of omega-3 fatty acids, which, if you don't eat oily fish, is a boon. It is also a complete protein, meaning it contains all nine essential amino acids required by the body. The seeds are also high in fibre, so they keep you full for longer. They make a perfect addition to energy balls, bars and snacks, since they are digested relatively slowly, providing slow-release energy and keeping blood sugar levels stable.

CHILLI/CHILE

A little fresh or dried chilli/chile can perk up a savoury or sweet energy snack, and works well with chocolate. Rich in vitamins C and E and carotenoids, chillies/chiles can help to relieve joint and muscle pain and have anti-inflammatory properties, so are perfect post-workout or if you're feeling achy.

COCONUT OIL

Over the last few years, coconut – in its many forms – has become hugely popular in the kitchen. When buying, do look for extra virgin or unrefined on the label, since refined versions are of poorer quality and nutritional value. Coconut oil contains a high proportion of medium-chain fatty acids, which are less likely to be stored as body fat and are a useful source of energy, although its high saturated fat content means it's best eaten in moderation. There's also evidence to suggest coconut is good for digestion, supporting the gut by destroying harmful bacteria, and helping the body to absorb fat-soluble vitamins and minerals.

FLAXSEEDS/LINSEEDS

Both ground and golden whole seeds are used in this book, particularly for their impressive range of health benefits unmatched by other types of seed. Most impressive is their heart- and brain-friendly omega-3 fatty acid content. This good fat supports the heart by protecting the blood vessels against inflammation. The seeds also provide antioxidant protection in the form of lignans, which improve cardiovascular health and the symptoms of the menopause by helping to redress hormone imbalance.

GARLIC

Part of the onion family, garlic has been prized for its health benefits for centuries and was used to maintain health and treat disease as far back as Egyptian times. While it contains a wide range of vitamins and minerals, it is garlic's sulphur, or more specifically allicin, content that provides significant benefits, protecting us from chronic diseases, certain cancers and heart disease. Garlic's antiviral, antifungal and antibacterial properties are most potent when eaten raw and, ideally, it should be eaten daily, chopped or minced, rather than sliced or the cloves left whole.

GINGER

This super-spice adds zing to your energy snacks and is excellent for digestion and gut health. An anti-inflammatory, ginger has been found to reduce the symptoms of, and pain associated with, arthritis and can help reduce exercise-induced muscle pain and soreness. All in all, it makes an excellent addition to post-exercise energy snacks.

GOJI BERRIES

These dried red berries have long been used in Chinese medicine to treat fatigue, high blood pressure and diabetes, and boost immunity. Vitamin C is found in generous amounts and the berries are also a good source of lutein, which benefits the eyes and is essential for healthy vision.

GUARANA

The powdered berry from this Amazonian plant has been found to be more energizing than caffeine-based drinks, including coffee, and so makes a perfect addition to an energy snack. Guarana stimulates the nervous system and, since it is released slowly in the body, it provides sustained long-term energy, helping to fight fatigue. It has quite a bitter taste, so is best used in moderation. It is also important to be mindful of recommended dosage and to check contraindications on the pack.

KEFIR

Numerous studies into this fermented milk product point to its incredible benefits to digestive and gut health, as well as potent antibacterial properties. Similar to yogurt in consistency, with a slightly sour taste, kefir can help to restore the balance of friendly bacteria in the gut and is also a good source of protein, B vitamins and calcium. It is easy to make your own using kefir grains – check online – or ready-made versions are increasingly available in health food shops and supermarkets.

LACUMA

Being naturally sweet with a slight caramel flavour, lacuma is useful when looking to reduce added sugar levels. It comes in powdered form and is a potent source of antioxidants, iron, calcium and vitamins B3 and C, and has anti-inflammatory properties.

MACA

Energy levels, strength and endurance are all said to benefit from this ancient Peruvian plant. With its lovely malty taste, maca adds flavour as well nutritional value to energy balls and other snacks, and as an adaptogen helps to support us when life is hectic, both physically and mentally. It is believed to benefit hormonal balance by supporting the endocrine system, which helps to regulate metabolism, sleep, mood, libido and fertility.

MATCHA

This vibrant green tea comes as a finely ground powder with impressively high antioxidant levels – one cup of matcha is said to contain as many antioxidants as ten cups of brewed green tea. These chemical compounds protect the body from free radical damage that can lead to cancer and other chronic diseases – not forgetting premature ageing. Other benefits are said to be enhanced mood, concentration and metabolism as well as weight loss, detoxification and an induced state of calm – an all-round winning combination!

NUTRITIONAL YEAST FLAKES

With a tangy cheesy flavour, nutritional yeast flakes – a great vegan alternative to dairy – make a worthy and convenient addition to the storecupboard. Don't be put off by their cumbersome name, the flakes add a welcome health boost to both raw and cooked savoury snacks, including B vitamins and minerals, such as iron, which are vital for energy production. The flakes are also a good plant source of protein, containing all the essential amino acids, and they are gluten-free.

POWDERED SUPER-GREENS

There are many super-green blends to choose from, but opt for a reputable brand containing a good range of nutrient-rich ingredients and in therapeutic quantities. A typical mix may feature an assortment of wheatgrass, chlorella, spirulina, alfalfa, barleygrass, vegetable powders, herbs and flaxseeds/ linseeds, providing a range of vitamins, minerals, phytonutrients, enzymes, antioxidants and fibre. The health benefits vary depending on the brand and it is possible to buy specific blends for energy-boosting, immunity support, detoxing and digestion.

PROTEIN POWDER

Protein is the building block of life and is essential for the repair and maintenance of every cell in the body. Plant protein powders are excellent as post-workout fuel and come in a readily digestible form, helping to speed recovery and energize the body. Look for pea-, hemp-, and soya-based powders.

QUINOA (GRAINS AND FLAKES)

Gluten-free and with twice the protein content of rice or barley, quinoa makes a great alternative to wheat and is a welcome addition to energy snacks. The grains need to be cooked first, but the flakes are fine enough to be used as they are in much the same way as you would rolled oats. Quinoa also contains useful amounts of omega-3 fatty acids and is high in anti-inflammatory phytonutrients.

SEA VEGETABLES

A valuable and familiar part of the Asian diet, the West has only relatively recently recognized the numerous health benefits of sea vegetables. Dried nori features in a number of recipes in this book and it provides a range of minerals, namely iodine, calcium, magnesium, potassium and iron. Sea vegetables in general help to boost immunity, aid metabolism and benefit the nervous system, reducing stress levels.

SPIRULINA

This blue-green algae is highly nutritious and has been found to have the ability to detoxify, regenerate and alkalize the body thanks to its rich chlorophyll content, which helps to transport oxygen to all cells in the body. But that's not all: the powder is rich in protein, iron, zinc and vitamins A, B, E and K, as well as phytonutrients – all in a readily usable and digestible form. Spirulina also supports the liver, kidneys, heart and digestive system. In this book, spirulina is largely interchangeable with wheatgrass or chlorella.

TURMERIC

The 'hot' spice of the moment, turmeric is an effective anti-inflammatory and has also been found to be antiviral and antibacterial, as well as containing a wealth of antioxidants. Curcumin is the active ingredient and it is more readily absorbed by the body if consumed with fat as well as piperine, a compound found in black pepper.

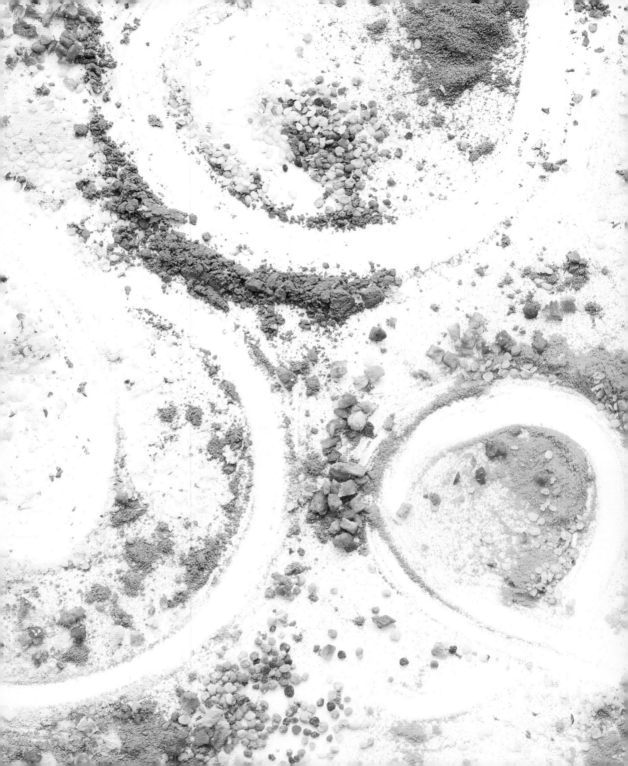

1

SUPERFOOD
RAW

BLUEBERRY BITES

Surprise… these purple-coloured, nutrient-rich balls have a fresh blueberry in the middle to give each one a burst of juicy freshness when bitten into. Purple foods are all the rage thanks to their immune-boosting abundance of antioxidants, particularly anthocyanins that play a protective role in the body.

40 g/1½ oz. almonds
1 tablespoon sunflower seeds
60 g/2¼ oz. unsweetened muesli base
1 small raw beetroot/beet, about 40 g/1½ oz., peeled and roughly chopped
60 g/2¼ oz. dried cranberries
3 tablespoons freshly squeezed orange juice
finely grated zest of ¼ unwaxed orange, plus extra to decorate
½ teaspoon ground cinnamon
2 teaspoons acai powder
8 fresh blueberries

MAKES 8

Put the almonds, sunflower seeds and muesli in a food processor and process for 2 minutes until very finely chopped. Add the beetroot, cranberries, orange juice, orange zest, cinnamon and acai powder, and blitz to a thick, smooth-ish paste, occasionally scraping down the mixture from the sides when needed.

With damp hands, take 1 tablespoon of the beetroot mixture and form into a round disc, then place a blueberry in the centre. Shape the mixture around the blueberry to make a ball about the size of a large walnut. Repeat to make 8 balls in total. Chill in the fridge for 30 minutes to firm up. Store in the fridge in an airtight container for up to 1 week. Decorate with a little extra orange zest to serve.

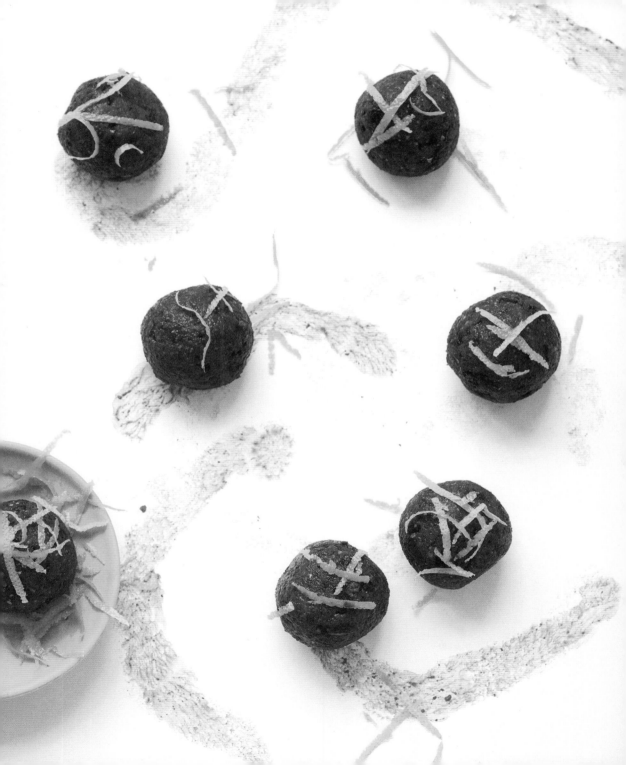

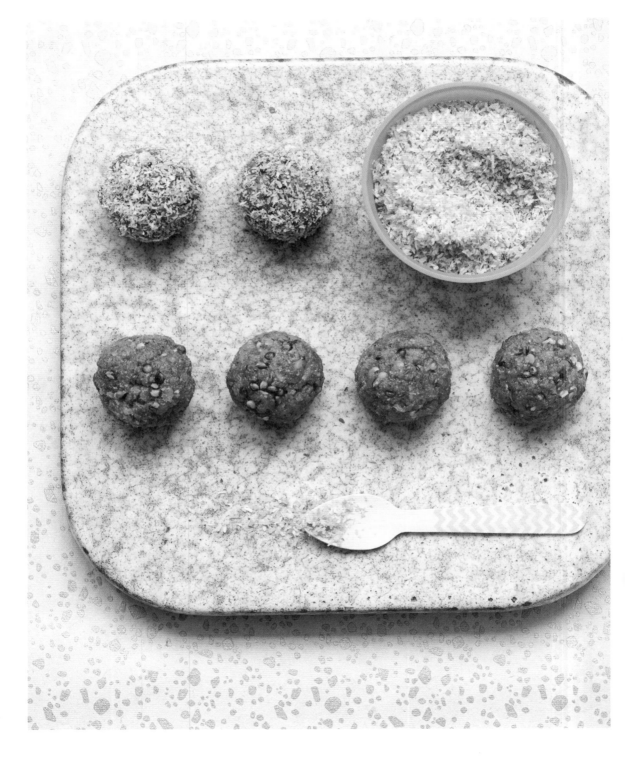

CARROT CAKE BALLS

If you can, choose soft, unsulphured apricots to make these balls, which are dark in colour with a lovely, sticky texture and toffee-like flavour. Sulphur is regularly used as a preservative in dried fruit and has been linked to exacerbating the symptoms of asthma. Hulled hemp seeds have a softer texture than the whole seeds and can be readily found in health food stores, larger supermarkets and online.

40 g/1½ oz. desiccated/dried unsweetened shredded coconut, for coating

25 g/1 oz. quinoa flakes or jumbo rolled oats

1 small carrot, about 50 g/1¾ oz., sliced

100 g/3½ oz. soft dried apricots, roughly chopped

1 tablespoon almond or cashew butter

1 teaspoon mixed/apple pie spice

1 tablespoon vanilla protein powder

1 tablespoon hulled hemp seeds

MAKES 8

First toast the desiccated/dried unsweetened shredded coconut. Place the coconut in a large, dry frying pan/skillet over a medium-low heat and cook for a couple of minutes, tossing the pan regularly, until light golden – take care as the coconut burns easily. Tip the toasted coconut onto a large plate and set aside while you make the balls.

Put the quinoa flakes (or oats) and carrot in a food processor and process until very finely chopped. Add the apricots, nut butter, mixed/apple pie spice and protein powder, and process again to a thick smooth-ish paste, occasionally scraping down the mixture from the sides when needed. Stir in the hemp seeds.

With damp hands, shape the carrot mixture into 8 large, walnut-sized balls, then roll each one in the toasted coconut until coated all over (any leftover coconut can be used in another recipe). Chill in the fridge for 30 minutes to firm up. Store in the fridge in an airtight container for up to 2 weeks.

BANANA BONANZA

Bananas are a great source of potassium, which regulates nerve and muscle function.

60 g/2¼ oz. roasted hazelnuts
70 g/2½ oz. jumbo rolled oats
1 large ripe banana, peeled
2 soft dried pitted dates, chopped
1 teaspoon pure vanilla extract
1 teaspoon ground cinnamon
2 teaspoons lacuma or maca powder
1 tablespoon cacao nibs
40 g/1½ oz. dried unsweetened banana chips
   (optional)

MAKES 10

Blitz the hazelnuts in a food processor until finely chopped, then add the oats and process again until everything is very finely chopped.

Next, add the banana, dates, vanilla, cinnamon and lacuma (or maca) powder, and process again to a thick, smooth-ish paste, occasionally scraping down the mixture from the sides when needed. Stir in the cacao nibs.

Using a mini food processor or grinder, blitz the banana chips, if using, until very finely chopped and tip them into a small bowl.

With damp hands, shape the banana mixture into 10 walnut-sized balls, then dunk each one in the chopped banana chips, if using, until coated all over. Chill for 30 minutes to firm up. Store in the fridge in an airtight container for up to 2 weeks.

AVO-CHOCO BALLS

These balls help keep you full for longer.

40 g/1½ oz. roasted hazelnuts, for coating
1 medium ripe avocado, cut in half and stone/pit
   removed
85 g/3 oz. soft dried pitted dates, roughly chopped
6 tablespoons ground almonds
1 tablespoon maple syrup or good-quality honey
4 tablespoons raw cacao powder, plus extra
   2 tablespoons for coating
1 teaspoon ground cinnamon
1 teaspoon pure vanilla extract

MAKES 10

Put the hazelnuts in a mini food processor or grinder and blitz until finely chopped, then set aside for coating.

Using a teaspoon, scoop the avocado flesh out of its skin into a food processor and add the rest of the ingredients. Blend to a thick, smooth-ish paste, occasionally scraping down the mixture from the sides when needed. If the mixture is very wet, add an extra tablespoon of cacao – you want it to be thick enough to hold together in a ball.

Put the remaining 2 tablespoons cacao powder in a bowl and stir in the blended hazelnuts.

With damp hands, shape the avocado mixture into 10 large marble-sized balls, then dunk each one in the cacao powder mixture until lightly coated all over. Chill for 30 minutes to firm up. Store in the fridge in an airtight container for up to 2 days.

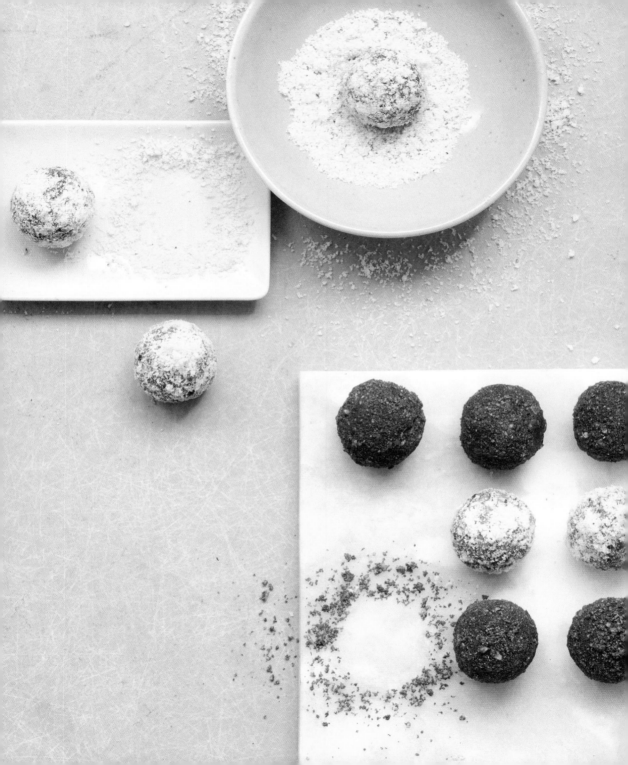

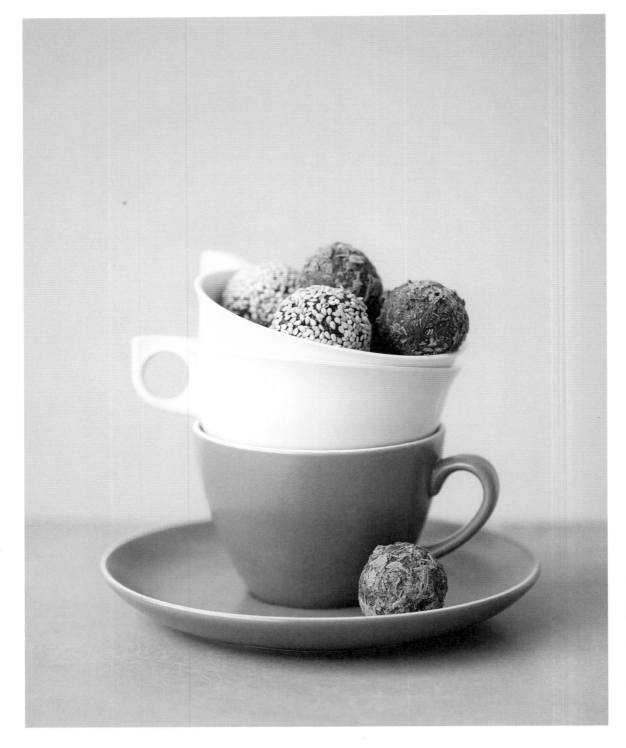

MORNING MOCHA

Feeling sluggish? These balls may be enough to perk you up.

50 g/1¾ oz. pecan nuts
50 g/1¾ oz. almonds
150 g/5½ oz. soft dried pitted dates, roughly chopped
3 tablespoons strong espresso coffee
2 tablespoons raw cacao nibs
1 tablespoon maca powder
40 g/1½ oz. dark/bittersweet (or raw) chocolate, 85% cocoa solids, finely grated, or raw cacao powder, for coating

MAKES 18

Toast the pecans in a large, dry frying pan/skillet over a medium-low heat for 3 minutes, turning once, until they start to colour. Tip the pecans into a food processor. Toast the almonds in the same way, then add to the food processor. Process for 2 minutes until the nuts start to form a paste, then scrape them into a mixing bowl.

Put the dates and coffee into the processor and blend to a thick paste, scraping down the mixture from the sides when needed. Spoon the mixture into the bowl containing the nuts and stir in the cacao nibs and maca.

Put the grated chocolate (or cacao powder) on a large plate. With damp hands, shape the mixture into 18 large, walnut-sized balls, then roll each one in the grated chocolate (or powder) until coated all over. Chill for 30 minutes to firm up. Store in the fridge in an airtight container for up to 2 weeks.

CHAI DATE BITES

A potent mix of herbal chai tea, turmeric and super-greens, these balls are a great source of antioxidants. They also help support the immune-system, digestion and fight inflammation in the body.

50 g/1¾ oz. pecan nuts
25 g/1 oz. sunflower seeds
100 g/3½ oz. soft dried pitted dates, chopped
1 tablespoon raw cacao powder
2 teaspoons herbal chai tea
½ teaspoon turmeric powder
2 teaspoons super-greens powder
3 tablespoons soy cream
25 g/1 oz. toasted sesame seeds, for coating

MAKES 10

Blitz the pecans and sunflower seeds in a food processor until very finely chopped. Add the dates and process to a thick, smooth-ish paste, occasionally scraping down the mixture from the sides when needed.

Add the cacao powder, chai tea, turmeric, super-greens powder and soy cream, and blend until combined.

Put the sesame seeds in a bowl.

With damp hands, shape the pecan mixture into 10 walnut-sized balls, then dunk each one in the sesame seeds until lightly coated all over. Chill for 30 minutes to firm up. Store in the fridge in an airtight container for up to 2 weeks.

LIME & MANGO BUZZ BALLS

A great alternative to caffeine, guarana helps to fight fatigue and provides sustained amounts of energy as it is released slowly in the body. From a tropical plant found in the Amazon, guarana has a slightly bitter flavour, so it is best used in moderation.

115 g/4 oz. dried mango pieces
50 g/1¾ oz. desiccated/dried
unsweetened shredded coconut
55 g/2 oz. Brazil nuts
finely grated zest of 2 unwaxed
limes
freshly squeezed juice of 1 lime
1 teaspoon guarana powder or chia
seeds
1 teaspoon bee pollen, for
sprinkling (optional)

MAKES 12

Put the mango in a heatproof bowl and pour over enough hot water to cover. Leave it to soak for 20 minutes until softened slightly but not completely rehydrated, then drain well and pat dry with paper towels.

While the mango is soaking, toast the coconut. Place the desiccated/dried unsweetened shredded coconut in a large, dry frying pan/skillet over a medium-low heat, then cook for a couple of minutes, tossing the pan regularly, until light golden – take care as the coconut burns easily.

Blitz the Brazils in a food processor until very finely chopped, then add the toasted coconut, softened mango, lime zest, lime juice and guarana powder (or chia seeds). Blend to a thick, smooth-ish paste, occasionally scraping down the mixture from the sides when needed.

With damp hands, shape the mango mixture into 12 walnut-sized balls, then sprinkle the tops with bee pollen, if you like. Chill for 30 minutes to firm up. Store in the fridge in an airtight container for up to 1 week.

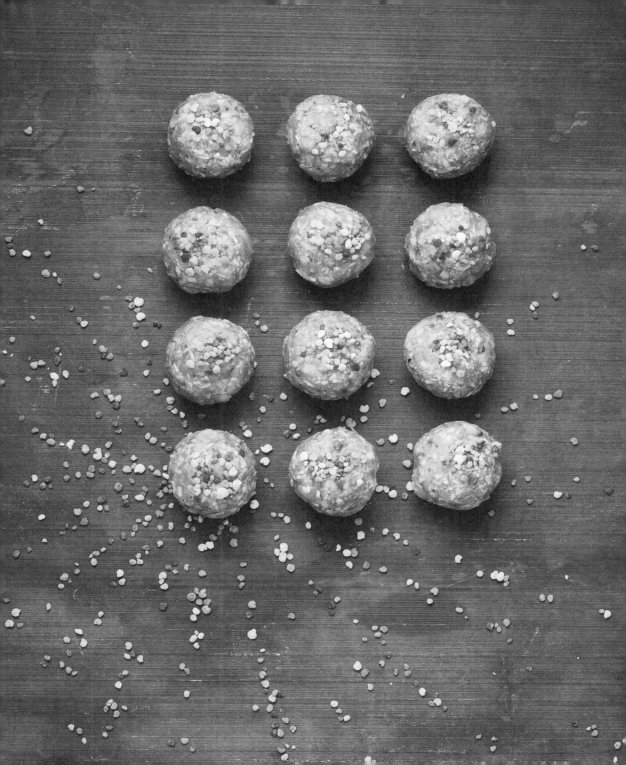

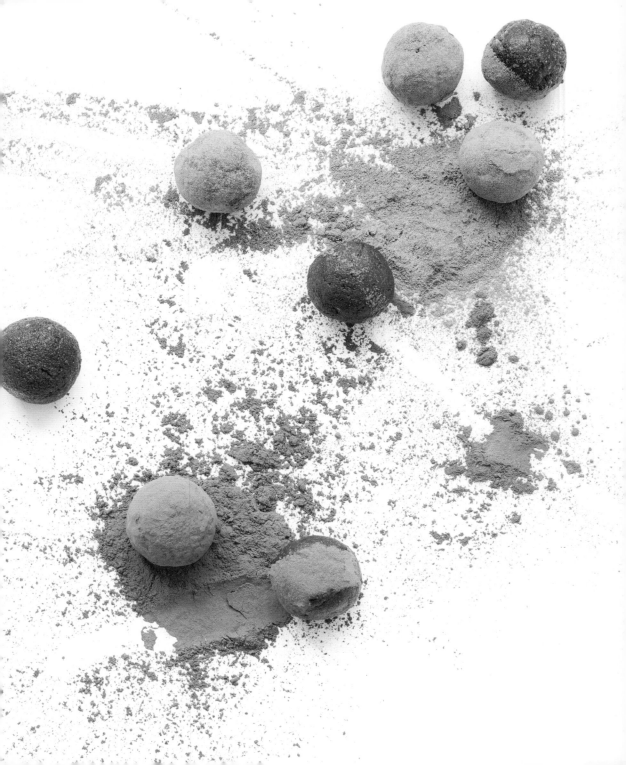

BEETROOT/BEET & CHOCOLATE BITES

Beetroot provides valuable nutrients including vitamin C, iron, potassium and fibre.

100 g/3½ oz. cashew nuts
40 g/1½ oz. quinoa flakes or jumbo rolled oats
70 g/2½ oz. peeled raw beetroot/beet, chopped
2 tablespoons raw cacao powder, plus extra for coating
2 tablespoons date syrup or good-quality honey
1 teaspoon pure vanilla extract
2 teaspoons spirulina, plus extra for sprinkling (optional)
1 tablespoon chia seeds
1 tablespoon almond milk

MAKES 10

Blitz the cashews in a food processor until finely chopped, then add the quinoa (or oats) and process again until very finely chopped. Tip the mixture into a mixing bowl.

Put the beetroot/beet in the processor and blitz to a coarse purée (use a blender if the quantity is too small for your processor). Spoon the purée into the mixing bowl and stir in the raw cacao powder, date syrup (or honey), vanilla, spirulina, chia seeds and almond milk.

Coat a plate with extra cacao powder. With damp hands, shape into 10 walnut-sized balls, then roll in cacao until lightly coated. Sprinkle a little spirulina over the top, if you like. Chill for 30 minutes to firm up. Store in the fridge in an airtight container for up to 2 weeks.

GREEN POWER BALLS

There are a number of super-greens powders around but most contain a base of spirulina, chlorella, wheatgrass and/or barley grass and are an effective way of getting a quick blast of nutrients into our bodies.

70 g/2½ oz. cashew nuts
25 g/1 oz. pumpkin seeds
40 g/1½ oz. quinoa flakes or jumbo rolled oats
1 tablespoon super-greens powder, plus extra for coating (optional)
100 g/3½ oz. soft dried pitted dates, roughly chopped
2 tablespoons almond milk

MAKES 10

Put the cashews, pumpkin seeds and quinoa flakes (or oats) in a food processor and process for a couple of minutes until very finely chopped and the oils start to release from the nuts.

Add the super-greens powder, dates and almond milk, and process again until the mixture forms a thick, coarse paste.

With damp hands, shape the cashew mixture into 10 large walnut-sized balls. If you like, generously coat a plate with extra super-greens powder and roll each ball until lightly coated all over, or alternatively leave them plain. Chill for 30 minutes to firm up. Store in the fridge in an airtight container for up to 2 weeks.

MATCHA & CARDAMOM BALLS

Brimming with antioxidants, matcha is perfect pre-workout as it is said to increase both energy levels and endurance. Memory and concentration also benefit – an excuse to have another ball in the afternoon, perhaps!

seeds from 4 cardamom pods
85 g/3 oz. shelled unsalted pistachios, plus extra 15 g/½ oz. for sprinkling
2 tablespoons pumpkin seeds
115 g/4 oz. soft dried figs, chopped
1 teaspoon coconut oil
2 teaspoons matcha powder, plus extra 2 teaspoons for sprinkling
1 tablespoon almond milk

MAKES 10

Using a pestle and mortar or spice grinder, grind the cardamom seeds to a powder, then set aside.

Put the pistachios and pumpkin seeds in a food processor and blitz until very finely chopped. Add the figs, coconut oil, matcha, almond milk and ground cardamom, and process to a thick, smooth-ish paste, occasionally scraping down the mixture from the sides when needed.

Finely chop the remaining pistachios for sprinkling.

With damp hands, shape the matcha mixture into 10 walnut-sized balls. Sprinkle a little matcha powder and chopped pistachios on top of each ball. Chill for 30 minutes to firm up. Store in the fridge in an airtight container for up to 2 weeks.

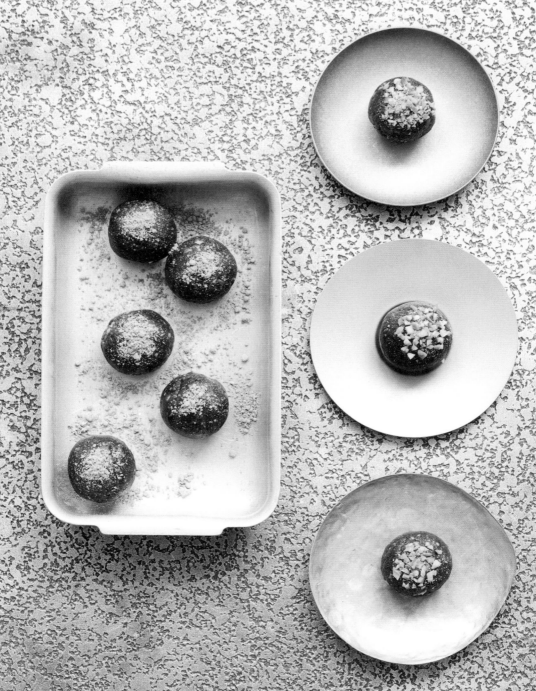

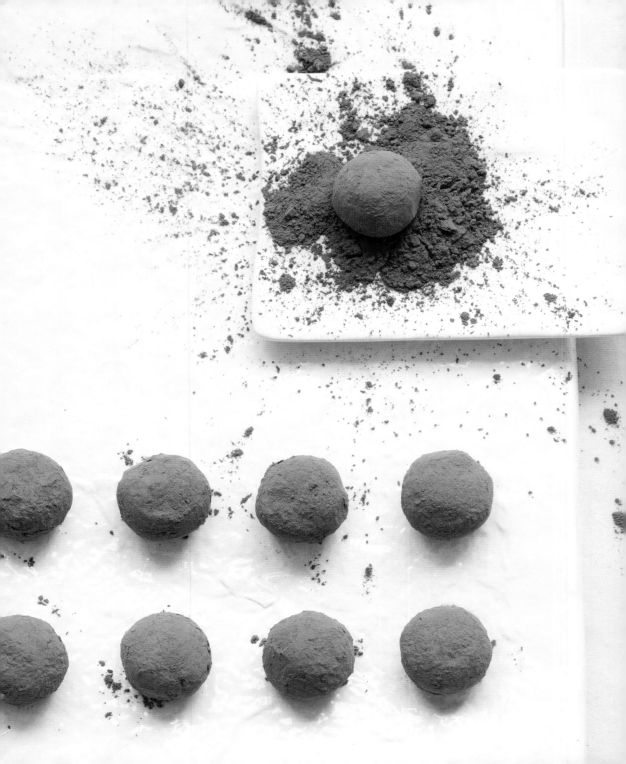

FIG, ORANGE & CARDAMOM BALLS

A classic combination of flavours that works beautifully together in an energy-packed ball. Cardamom lends more than just flavour, being good for digestion, nausea, bloating and lack of appetite.

seeds from 3 cardamom pods
50 g/1¾ oz. almonds
50 g/1¾ oz. cashew nuts
100 g/3½ oz. soft dried figs,
  roughly chopped
3 tablespoons freshly squeezed
  orange juice
finely grated zest of ½ unwaxed
  orange
3 tablespoons raw cacao powder,
  plus extra for coating

MAKES 12

Using a pestle and mortar, grind the cardamom seeds until very finely ground, then set aside.

Put the almonds and cashews in a food processor and process for 2 minutes until the nuts start to form a coarse paste, then scrape them into a bowl.

Add the figs to the food processor and process to a thick paste, occasionally scraping down the mixture from the sides when needed. Return the ground nuts to the processor with the orange juice, orange zest, raw cacao and ground cardamom seeds, then blend until combined.

Generously coat a plate with extra cacao powder.

With damp hands, shape the fig mixture into 12 large walnut-sized balls, then roll each one in the cacao powder until lightly coated all over. Chill for 30 minutes to firm up. Store in the fridge in an airtight container for up to 2 weeks.

BERRY BOUNTY
BALLS

Acai berries (and the freeze-dried powder) have impressive nutritional properties and are good post-exercise, helping to boost energy levels, support the immune system and aid digestive health. As an added bonus, berries are great for the brain and have been found to help stave off age-related memory decline.

50 g/1¾ oz. cashew nuts
100 g/3½ oz. dried blueberries
50 g/1¾ oz. fresh blueberries
40 g/1½ oz. desiccated/dried unsweetened shredded coconut
1 tablespoon ground flaxseeds/ linseeds
1 tablespoon hulled hemp seeds
1 tablespoon acai powder
2 teaspoons raw cacao powder, for coating

MAKES 12

Put the cashews in a food processor and process until very finely chopped.

Add the dried and fresh blueberries, coconut and ground flaxseeds/linseeds and process again to a thick, smooth-ish paste, occasionally scraping down the mixture from the sides when needed. Stir in the hemp seeds and the acai powder.

Put the cacao powder on a plate.

With damp hands, shape the blueberry mixture into 12 walnut-sized balls, then dunk one half of each ball into the cacao powder until coated. Chill for 30 minutes to firm up. Store in the fridge in an airtight container for up to 1 week.

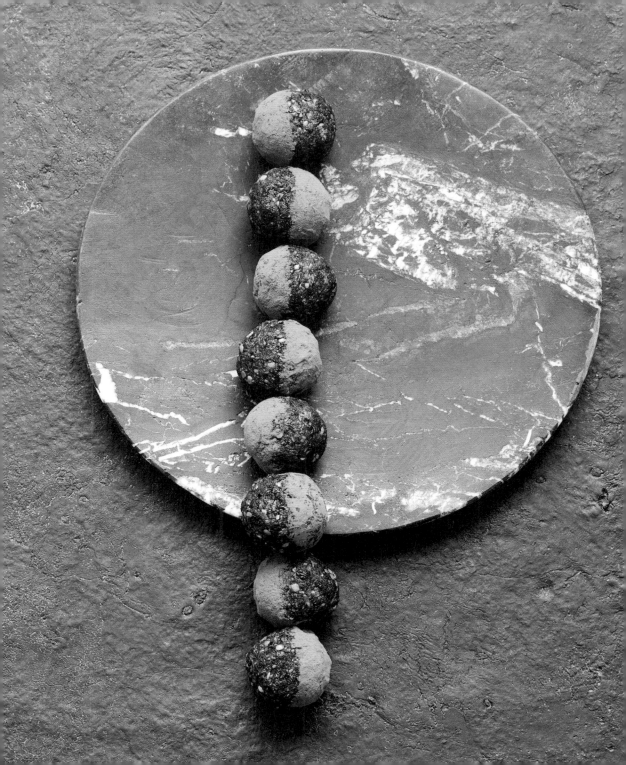

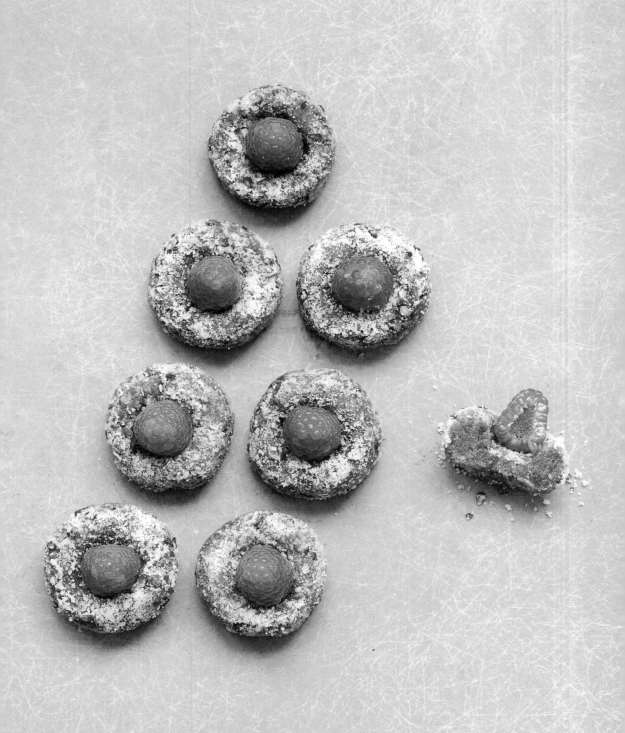

DOUBLE RASPBERRY MACA BALLS

A delicious combination of fresh and dried raspberries, butterscotch-flavoured maca, vanilla and creamy nuts. Since the balls contain fresh fruit, they don't have as long a shelf-life as those made purely with dried, around a week, but they are sure to be snapped up before that.

100 g/3½ oz. cashew nuts

2–3 tablespoons ground almonds, plus extra 1 tablespoon for coating

1 tablespoon maca powder

2 teaspoons pure vanilla extract

100 g/3½ oz. soft dried pitted dates, roughly chopped

60 g/2¼ oz. fresh raspberries, plus extra 10 to decorate

1 tablespoon freeze-dried raspberries, plus extra 2 tablespoons for coating

MAKES 10

Put the cashews in a food processor and process for a couple of minutes until very finely chopped and the oils start to release from the nuts.

Add 2 tablespoons of the ground almonds, the maca powder, vanilla, dates and fresh raspberries to the processor and blitz to a thick, smooth-ish paste, occasionally scraping down the mixture from the sides when needed. If the mixture is very wet, add a further 1 tablespoon of ground almonds, then stir in the freeze-dried raspberries.

Mix together the ground almonds for coating with the remaining freeze-dried raspberries for coating on a plate.

With damp hands, shape the raspberry mixture into 10 large walnut-sized balls, then roll each one in the almond and raspberry mixture. Take one ball and press it down slightly with your thumb into a flattened round with a dip in the middle. Place a raspberry in the dip, then repeat with the remaining balls and raspberries. Chill for 30 minutes to firm up. Store in the fridge in an airtight container for up to 3 days.

PASSION FRUIT ZOOM BITES

Just the thing to get you going in the morning… the passion fruit adds wonderful flavour and colour, not forgetting an abundance of immune-boosting vitamin C.

100 g/3½ oz. almonds or macadamia nuts
100 g/3½ oz. soft dried apricots, chopped
1 teaspoon pure vanilla extract
2 tablespoons desiccated/dried unsweetened shredded coconut, plus extra for sprinkling
1 tablespoon vanilla protein powder
1 teaspoon coconut oil
2 passion fruit, cut in half

brownie pan, lined with clingfilm/plastic wrap

MAKES 10

Blitz the almonds (or macadamia) in a food processor until very finely ground. Add three-quarters of the apricots along with the vanilla, coconut, protein powder and coconut oil.

Using a teaspoon, scoop out the passion fruit pulp and add to the processor. Blend to a thick, smooth-ish paste, occasionally scraping down the mixture from the sides when needed.

Finely chop the remaining apricots and stir them into the mixture.

Spoon the apricot mixture into the lined brownie pan and spread it out with the back of a damp spoon into an even layer about 1 cm/½ inch thick. Sprinkle a little extra coconut over the top. Chill for 30 minutes to firm up, then cut into 10 pieces. Store in the fridge in an airtight container for up to 1 week.

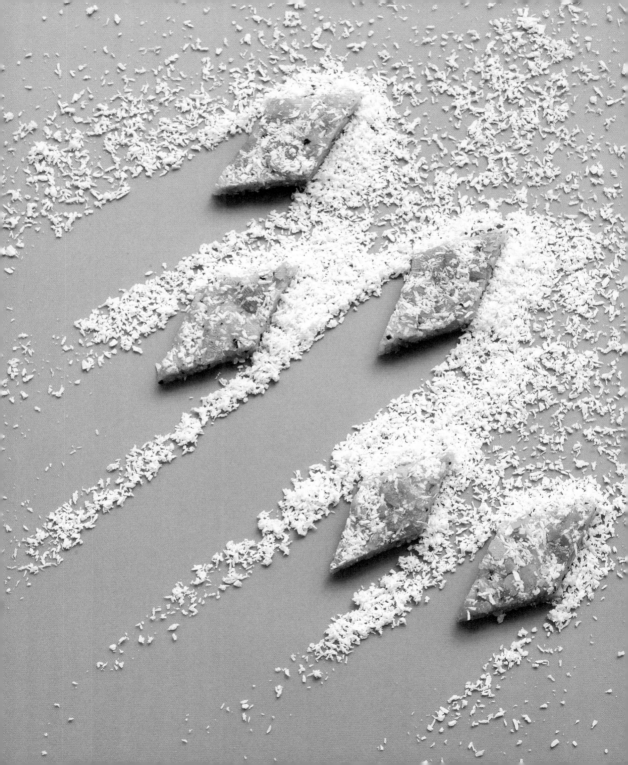

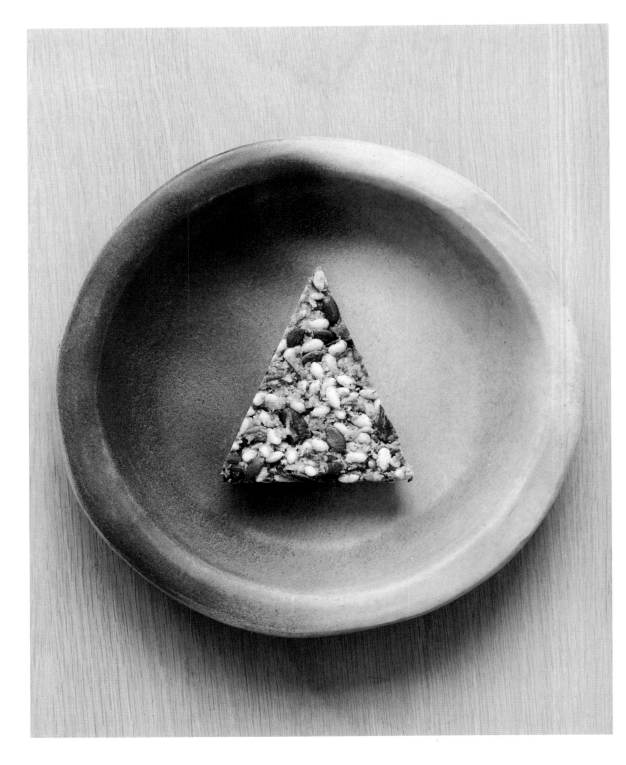

NO-BAKE
BREAKFAST BARS

The pecans and coconut are pan-toasted first before combining with the rest of the ingredients. This step isn't essential but it does give these nut- and seed-rich bars an extra level of flavour.

100 g/3½ oz. pecan nuts
40 g/1½ oz. wholegrain
   unsweetened puffed rice
40 g/1½ oz. porridge oats
60 g/2¼ oz. pumpkin seeds
2 tablespoons ground flaxseeds/
   linseeds
1 tablespoon chia seeds
1 teaspoon ground cinnamon
pinch of sea salt
50 g/1¾ oz. desiccated/dried
   unsweetened shredded coconut
75ml/2½ fl oz. maple syrup
40 g/1½ oz. coconut oil
125 g/4½ oz. peanut butter
   (smooth or crunchy)

20-cm/8-inch baking pan, lined with clingfilm/plastic wrap, leaving enough overhang to cover the top

MAKES 12

Put the pecan nuts in a large, dry frying pan/skillet and toast over a medium-low heat for 4 minutes, turning once, until they start to colour and smell toasted. Tip the nuts into a bowl and leave to cool and crisp up.

Meanwhile, put the puffed rice, oats, pumpkin seeds, flaxseeds/linseeds, chia seeds and cinnamon in a mixing bowl. Add the pinch of salt.

Once the pecans are toasted and cooling, tip the coconut into the frying pan/skillet and toast for a couple of minutes; keep an eye on it as it can easily burn. Tip the coconut into the mixing bowl with the puffed rice mixture. Break the pecans into large pieces and add to the mixing bowl and stir until everything is combined.

Gently heat the maple syrup and coconut oil in a small pan until melted. Remove from the heat and stir in the peanut butter. Pour the mixture into the dry ingredients and stir well until combined.

Tip the mixture into the prepared pan and spread it out into an even layer using the back of a spoon (it helps to dampen the spoon). Fold the overhanging clingfilm/plastic wrap over the top and chill in the fridge for at least an hour (or in the freezer for 30 minutes). When firm, lift out of the pan using the clingfilm/plastic wrap to help, then cut into 12 bars. Store in an airtight container for up to 1 week.

CHOCOLATE GOJI BARS

Packed with nuts, seeds, wholegrains and dried fruit, these moreish cereal bars couldn't be easier to make. Do add your own combinations of ingredients – just keep the proportions the same.

175 g/6 oz. good-quality honey
3 tablespoons coconut oil
3 tablespoons almond butter
100 g/3½ oz. toasted hazelnuts, roughly chopped
55 g/2 oz. sunflower seeds
2 tablespoons hulled hemp seeds
40 g/1½ oz. wholegrain unsweetened puffed rice
90 g/3¼ oz. jumbo rolled oats
60 g/2¼ oz. goji berries
40 g/1½ oz. raw cacao powder
pinch of sea salt

25 x 20-cm/10 x 8-inch baking pan, lined with clingfilm/plastic wrap, leaving enough overhang to cover the top

MAKES 18

Gently heat the honey and coconut oil in a small pan until melted. Remove from the heat and stir in the almond butter.

Mix together the rest of the ingredients in a mixing bowl. Add the honey mixture and stir until combined.

Tip the puffed rice mixture into the lined pan and spread out into an even layer with the back of a damp spoon, pressing it down into a firm, even layer. Fold over the overhanging clingfilm/plastic wrap to cover the top of the mixture, then chill for 1 hour to firm up. Cut into 18 bars and keep stored in the fridge in an airtight container for up to 1 week.

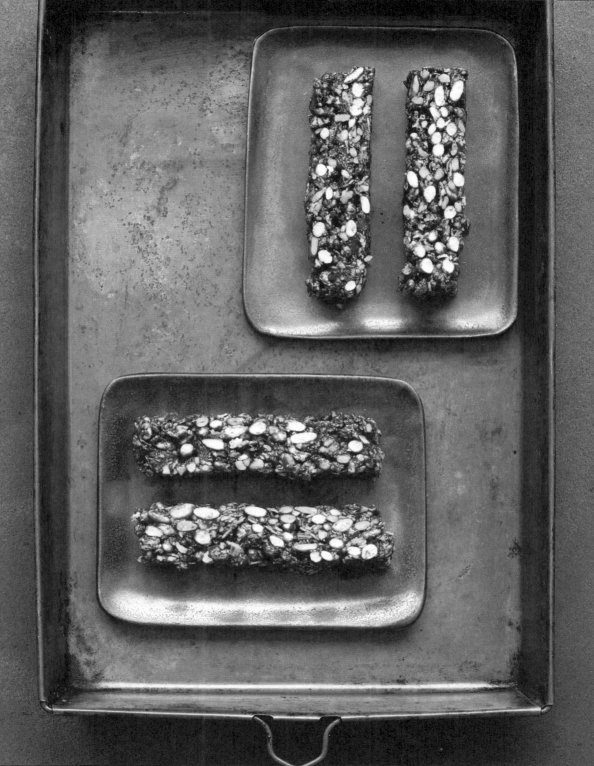

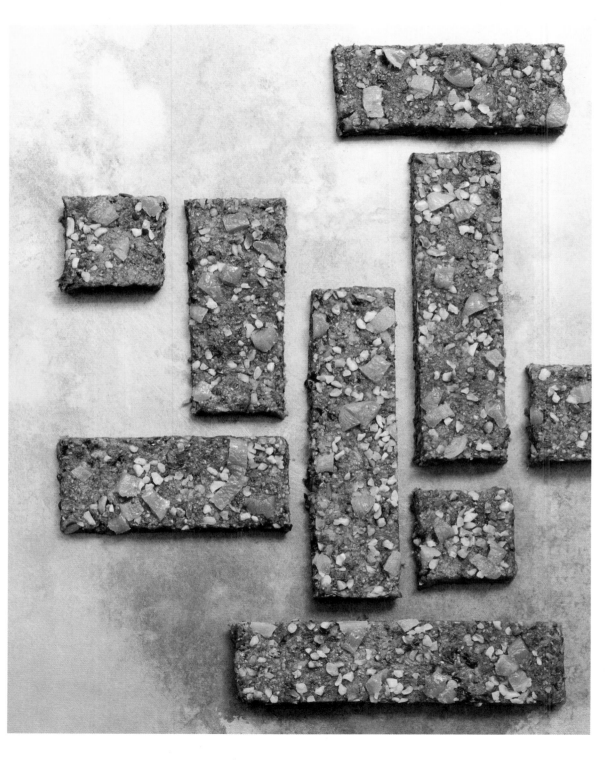

SPICED FRUIT BARS

A healthful combination of dried fruits, oats, nuts, seeds and naturally sweet spices – and, yes, veg – these bars are perfect for sustaining energy levels and giving you a boost pre- or post-exercise. Particularly noteworthy is the bone protective capabilities of prunes. Research has found that eating prunes on a regular basis can both prevent and reverse bone loss.

115 g/4 oz. roasted hazelnuts, roughly chopped
40 g/1½ oz. jumbo rolled oats
125 g/4½ oz. pitted dried prunes, chopped
70 g/2½ oz. soft dried apricots, chopped
1 tablespoon chia seeds
2 teaspoons mixed/apple pie spice
1 carrot, about 50 g/1¾ oz., finely grated
2 tablespoons pumpkin seeds, roughly chopped
finely grated zest and freshly squeezed juice of 1 large unwaxed orange

baking pan, lined with clingfilm/ plastic wrap

MAKES 16

Put 100 g/3½ oz. of the hazelnuts in a food processor and blitz until finely chopped, then add the oats and process again until everything is very finely chopped.

Add the prunes and 50 g/1¾ oz. of the apricots and process to a thick, smooth-ish paste, occasionally scraping down the mixture from the sides when needed. Stir in the chia seeds, mixed/apple pie spice, carrot, pumpkin seeds, orange zest and orange juice.

Spoon the fruit mixture into the lined baking pan and spread out with the back of a dampened spoon until it is about 1 cm/½ inch thick.

Cut the remaining apricots into small pieces and scatter over the top. Repeat with the rest of the hazelnuts, pressing the nuts and apricots down slightly to help them stick to the fruit mixture. Chill for 30 minutes to firm up, then cut into 16 bars, each 2 cm/¾ inch wide. Store in the fridge in an airtight container for up to 2 weeks.

LEMON BLISS BITES

These coconut and cacao butter bites are given an extra lemony kick thanks to the addition of finely grated lemon zest. As the zest is used, do look for unwaxed fruit. Citrus fruit is routinely coated in a protective wax, which is often plastic-based, to protect the fruit in transit and extend its shelf life. If you can't find unwaxed lemons, scrub the fruit well under hot running water to remove it, then pat dry.

25 g/1 oz. desiccated/dried unsweetened shredded coconut, plus 2 tablespoons for sprinkling
85 g/3 oz. cashew nuts
15 g/½ oz. raw cacao butter or creamed coconut, cut into small pieces
1 tablespoon good-quality honey
4 teaspoons vanilla protein powder
finely grated zest and juice of 1 large unwaxed lemon
a handful of goji berries

baking pan, lined with clingfilm/plastic wrap

MAKES 8–10

First toast the desiccated/dried unsweetened shredded coconut, including the extra coconut for sprinkling over the bites at the end. Place the coconut in a large, dry frying pan/skillet over a medium-low heat, then cook for a couple of minutes, tossing the pan regularly, until light golden – take care as the coconut burns easily. If preferred, leave the desiccated/dried unsweetened shredded coconut untoasted.

Set aside 2 tablespoons of the toasted coconut and tip the remaining coconut into a food processor with the cashews, cacao butter (or creamed coconut), honey, protein powder, lemon zest and lemon juice. Process to a thick, smooth-ish paste, occasionally scraping down the mixture from the sides when needed.

Spoon the lemon mixture into the lined pan (or form into 8 balls). Using the back of a wet spoon, spread into an even layer, about 1.5 cm/⅝ inch thick, then cut into 8–10 squares. Scatter the reserved toasted coconut and the goji berries over the top, pressing them down slightly to help them stick. If making balls, roll each ball in the reserved toasted coconut and place a goji berry on top. Chill for 30 minutes to firm up. Store in the fridge in an airtight container for up to 2 weeks.

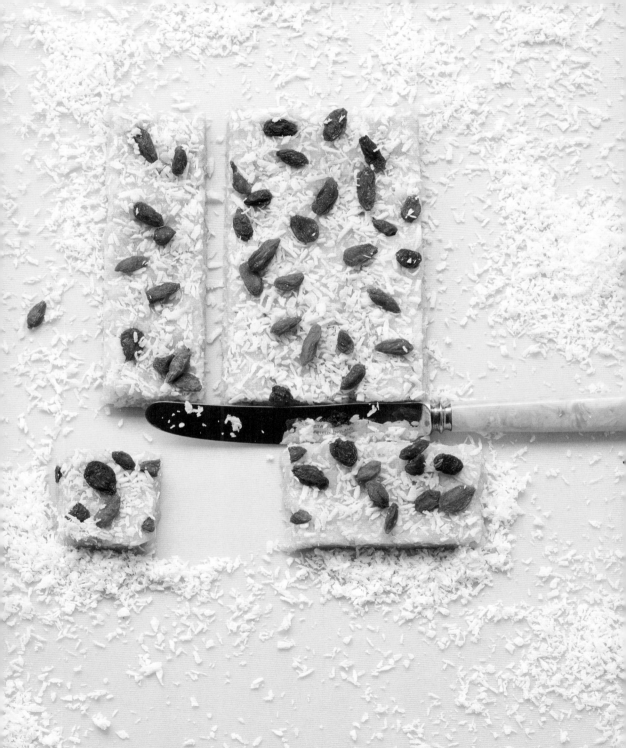

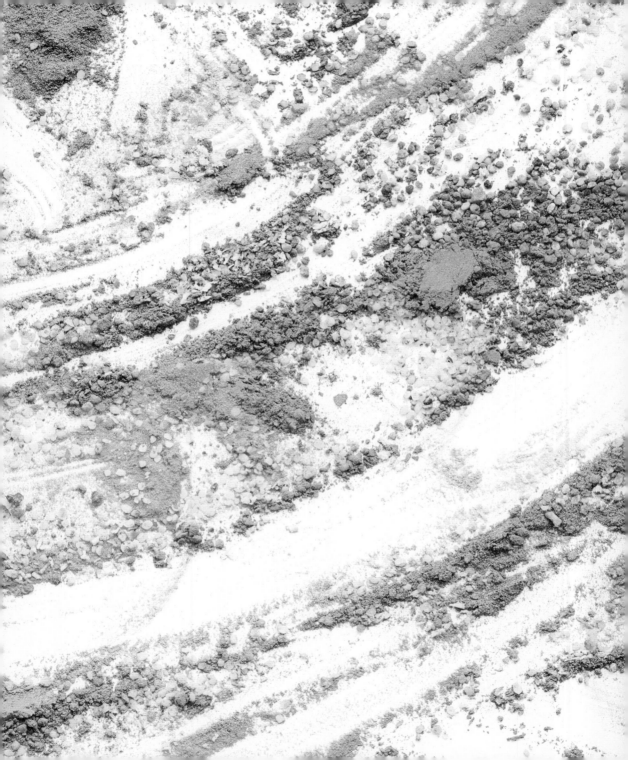

2

SUPERFOOD
COOKED

APPLE CRUMBLIES

With all the flavour of a traditional apple crumble, these fruity flapjack-style bars make a delicious afternoon treat. Apple – and there's a double dose of the fruit in these – may help to boost exercise endurance and performance thanks to its quercetin content. This antioxidant improves lung efficiency as well as boosting the immune system.

90 g/3¼ oz. maple syrup
4 tablespoons coconut oil, plus extra for greasing
175 g/6 oz. jumbo rolled oats
60 g/2¼ oz. pecan nuts
50 g/1¾ oz. pumpkin seeds
1 tablespoon chia seeds
2 teaspoons mixed spice/apple pie spice
50 g/1¾ oz. dried apples, roughly chopped
1 small eating apple, cored and grated (no need to peel)
2 eggs, lightly beaten
1 teaspoon pure vanilla extract

23-cm/9-inch baking pan, base lined with baking parchment and sides greased

MAKES 12–16

Preheat the oven to 180°C (350°F) Gas 4.

Gently heat the maple syrup and coconut oil in a saucepan.

Meanwhile, put the oats, pecans, pumpkin seeds, chia seeds and mixed spice/apple pie spice in a mixing bowl and stir well until combined. Add the dried and freshly grated apples. Beat the eggs with the vanilla, add to the bowl and mix together.

Spoon the apple mixture into the prepared pan and spread it out into an even layer, pressing down firmly with the back of a wet spoon.

Bake for 30–35 minutes until firmed up and light golden; it will crisp up further when cool. Leave to cool in the pan, then lift out, using the baking parchment to help you, and cut into 12–16 pieces. Store in an airtight container for 3–5 days.

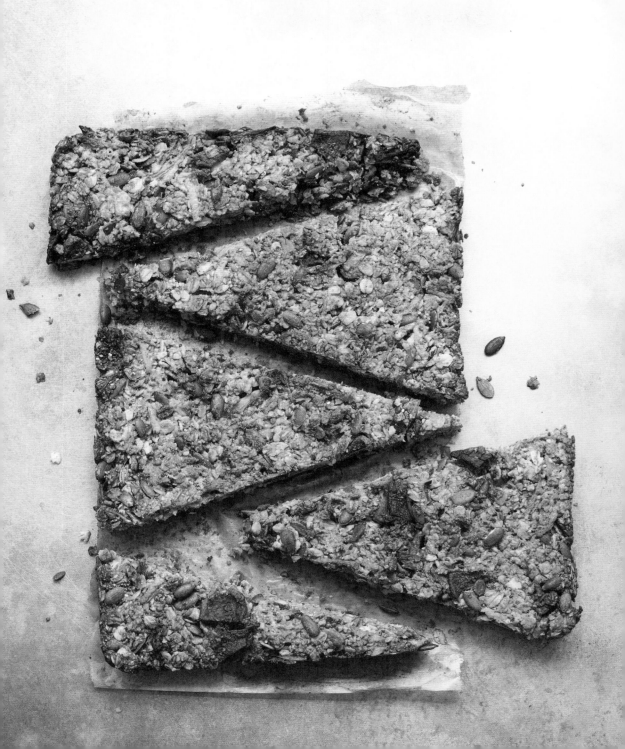

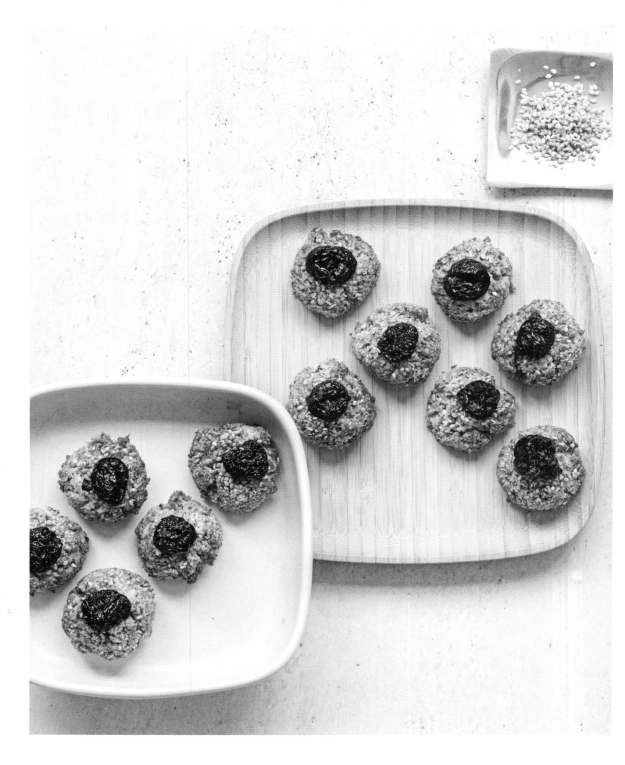

COCONUT & CHERRY DROPS

Similar to coconut macaroons, these come with a health boost thanks to the addition of ground flaxseeds/linseeds and sesame seeds. Despite their diminutive size, flaxseeds/linseeds are a good source of omega-3 fatty acids, while sesame seeds provide a range of minerals, including zinc, calcium, magnesium and iron.

85 g/3 oz. desiccated/dried unsweetened shredded coconut
25 g/1 oz. coconut sugar
1 tablespoon ground flaxseeds/ linseeds
25 g/1 oz. ground almonds
2 egg whites
1 teaspoon toasted sesame seeds
14 dried sour cherries

baking sheet, lined with baking parchment

MAKES 14

Preheat the oven to 180°C (350°F) Gas 4.

Mix together the coconut, coconut sugar, ground flaxseeds/linseeds and ground almonds in a bowl.

Whisk the egg whites in a grease-free mixing bowl until they form soft peaks. Gently fold the coconut mixture into the egg whites one-third at a time, taking care not to lose too much air, until incorporated.

Using a tablespoon, place rounded scoops of the mixture onto the prepared baking sheet. Sprinkle with a few sesame seeds and place a cherry on top of each one. Bake for 10–12 minutes until golden and firm. Leave to cool on the baking sheet for 5 minutes before transferring to a wire rack to cool completely. The coconut drops will keep stored in an airtight container for up to 3 days.

DOUBLE-GINGER-NUT BITES

These bite-sized snacks come with a double dose of ginger, which not only adds a flavour boost but also provides valuable medicinal properties. Ginger has long been revered for being good for the digestive system, however, it is also a potent anti-inflammatory so can help those with osteoarthritis or rheumatoid arthritis – rather like its botanical family member, turmeric.

125 g/4½ oz. soft dried apricots, chopped
2 tablespoons maple syrup
2 tablespoons coconut oil
90 g/3¼ oz. rolled oats
1 teaspoon ground ginger
2-cm/¾-inch piece of fresh root ginger, peeled and finely grated
20 g/¾ oz. pecan nuts, roughly chopped

baking sheet, lined with baking parchment

MAKES 14

Preheat the oven to 180°C (350°F) Gas 4.

Put the apricots in a small pan with 6 tablespoons of water and cook, covered, over a low heat until softened, occasionally crushing the apricots with the back of a fork to break them down. This should take 8–10 minutes; the water will be fully absorbed by the fruit.

Transfer the apricots to a blender with the maple syrup and coconut oil, and blend until puréed.

Mix the oats together with the ground ginger, fresh ginger and pecans in a mixing bowl. Stir in the apricot purée until combined.

With damp hands, shape the apricot mixture into 14 walnut-sized balls and place them on the prepared baking sheet. Using your fingers, press down on the top of each ball to flatten to about 1 cm/½ inch thick.

Bake for 15–20 minutes until slightly golden around the edges, then transfer to a wire rack to cool. Store in an airtight container for 3–5 days.

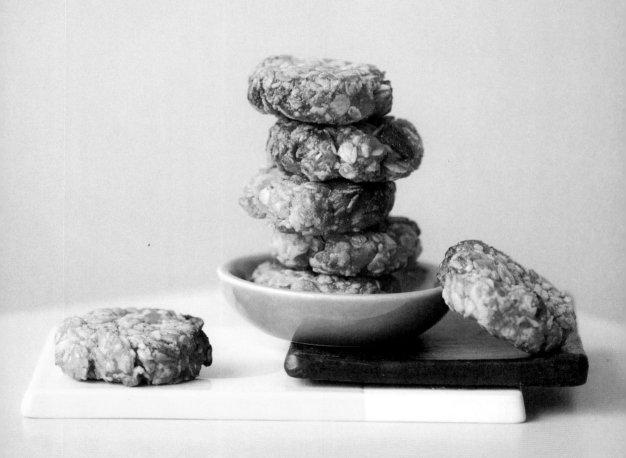

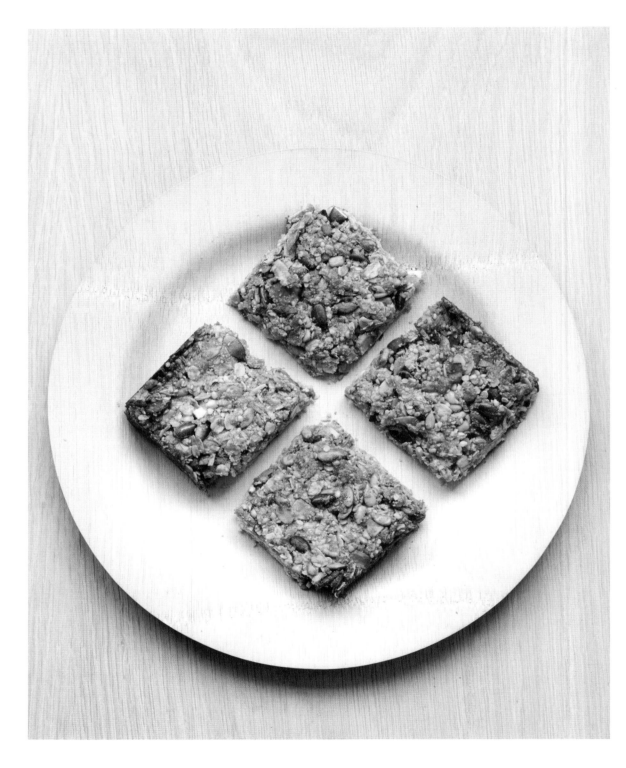

HEMP PROTEIN SQUARES

Packed with nuts and seeds, these bars contain hulled hemp seeds, which are bursting with a perfectly balanced combination of heart-friendly essential fatty acids omega-3 and omega-6. They also contain protein in a more readily digestible form than meat and dairy products.

55 g/2 oz. blanched hazelnuts
100 g/3½ oz. cashew nuts
140 g/5 oz. jumbo rolled/old-fashioned oats
40 g/1½ oz. unsweetened flaked coconut
70 g/2½ oz. pumpkin seeds, roughly chopped
70 g/2½ oz. sunflower seeds
4 tablespoons hulled hemp seeds
1½ teaspoons ground cinnamon
pinch of sea salt
4 tablespoons coconut oil
100ml/3½ fl oz. good-quality honey
2 teaspoons pure vanilla extract

23-cm/9-inch baking pan, lined with baking parchment

MAKES 16

Preheat the oven to 180°C (350°F) Gas 4.

Place the hazelnuts and cashews on a baking sheet and toast for 10 minutes, tossing the nuts halfway through, until they start to turn light golden. Remove from the oven and tip them into a food processor.

Place the oats on a second baking sheet and toast at the same time as the nuts for 5 minutes until they start to colour. Tip them into the food processor with the nuts, then blitz until coarsely chopped.

Once the nuts are roasted, place the flaked coconut on the baking sheet in the oven for 4 minutes until it starts to turn golden. Tip the coconut into a bowl and crush it a little with your hands. Add the nut and oat mixture, the three types of seeds, the cinnamon and pinch of salt.

Gently heat the coconut oil and honey in a pan until melted. Stir in the vanilla and pour into the nut mixture. Stir until everything is mixed together thoroughly, then tip the mixture into the prepared pan. Press down into a firm even layer with the back of a dampened spoon. Bake for 20–25 minutes until golden and firm. Mark into 16 squares and leave in the pan for 10 minutes before lifting out, using the baking parchment to help you. Separate into squares and leave to cool on a wire rack. Store in an airtight container for 3–5 days.

BANANA
OAT BITES

These contain no added sugar, deriving their natural sweetness from bananas and dates. They require very little effort to make and therefore are perfect for an afternoon boost when energy levels may need perking up.

40 g/1½ oz. pecan nuts
2 ripe bananas, peeled and
chopped
2 teaspoons coconut oil, melted
1 teaspoon pure vanilla extract
90 g/3¼ oz. jumbo rolled oats
2 teaspoons chia seeds
¼ teaspoon sea salt
4 soft dried pitted dates, chopped
1 teaspoon ground cinnamon

baking sheet, lined with baking
parchment

MAKES 10

Preheat the oven to 180°C (350°F) Gas 4.

Toast the pecans in a large, dry frying pan/skillet for 4 minutes, turning once, until they start to colour. Leave to cool, then roughly chop.

Mash the bananas in a mixing bowl to a smooth purée. Stir in all the remaining ingredients and toasted pecans and stir until combined.

Place heaped tablespoonfuls of the mixture onto the prepared baking sheet; the mixture will make around 10. Press down each bite with your fingers into a round about 1 cm/½ inch thick. Bake for 20–25 minutes until golden and crisp.

Leave to cool for 5 minutes before transferring to a wire rack to cool completely. They will keep stored in an airtight container for up to 5 days.

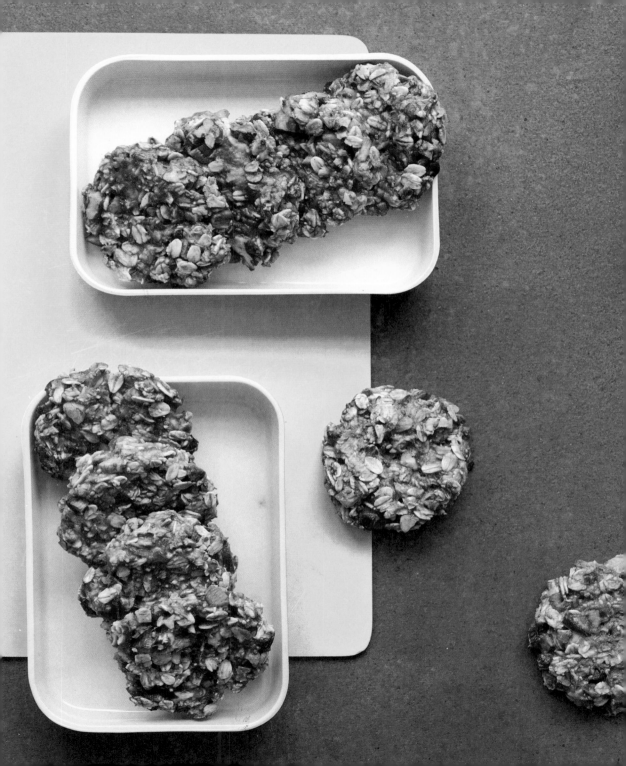

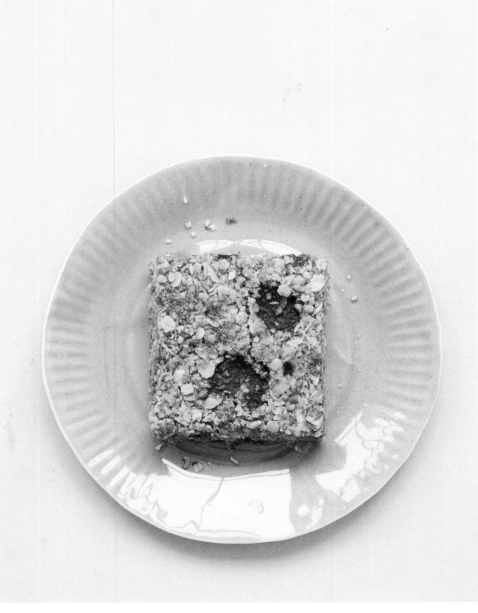

RASPBERRY, COCONUT & LEMON BARS

These are erring on the side of being a treat, rather than an everyday energy bar. They have a slightly softer texture than, say, a flapjack, and the fresh raspberries and lemon add a zingy note. Coconut sugar can be found in health food shops and online and has a lovely, deep caramel flavour. Nutritionally, being unrefined, it retains some of its antioxidants, vitamins, minerals and fibre. However, do eat it in moderation – it's still a type of sugar.

100 g/3½ oz. hazelnuts, roughly chopped
100 g/3½ oz. rolled/old-fashioned oats
100 g/3½ oz. wholemeal/ whole-wheat spelt flour
90 g/3¼ oz. coconut sugar
50 g/1¾ oz. desiccated/dried unsweetened shredded coconut
finely grated zest and freshly squeezed juice of
1 large unwaxed lemon
125 g/4½ oz. coconut oil
140 g/5 oz. frozen raspberries

23-cm/9-inch baking pan, lined with baking parchment

MAKES 16

Preheat the oven to 190°C (375°F) Gas 5.

Put three-quarters of the hazelnuts in a food processor and process until very finely chopped. Set aside the remaining chopped hazelnuts.

Put the finely chopped hazelnuts, oats, flour, coconut sugar, desiccated/dried unsweetened shredded coconut and lemon zest in a mixing bowl.

Gently melt the coconut oil over a low heat, then pour it into the bowl with the lemon juice. Stir until combined, then gently fold in the raspberries. Transfer the mixture to the prepared pan and scatter over the reserved chopped hazelnuts.

Bake for 35–40 minutes, or until firm and light golden. Leave to cool completely in the pan, then lift out, using the baking parchment to help you, and cut into 16 squares. Store in an airtight container for 3–5 days.

CHOC-CHIP QUINOA BARS

Quinoa flakes can be found in health food shops or online and are more delicate in texture than oats – that said, they are interchangeable in this recipe. Healthwise, quinoa is a complete protein meaning it contains all nine amino acids required by the body, it's high in fibre and also contains good levels of vitamins B and E along with some omega-3 fatty acids. Flaxseeds/linseeds also are brimming with the latter.

90 g/3¼ oz. walnuts, roughly chopped
3 tablespoons hulled hemp seeds
90 g/3¼ oz. flaxseeds/linseeds
5 tablespoons raw cacao nibs
4 tablespoons quinoa flakes or rolled/old-fashioned oats
¼ teaspoon sea salt
200 g/7 oz. soft dried pitted dates, chopped
115 g/4 oz. peanut butter

25 x 20-cm/10 x 8-inch baking pan, lined with baking parchment

MAKES 16

Preheat the oven to 180°C (350°F) Gas 4.

Blitz half of the walnuts, hemp seeds and flaxseeds/linseeds in a food processor until finely ground. Tip into a mixing bowl and mix with the remaining walnuts, hemp seeds, flaxseeds/linseeds, cacao nibs, quinoa flakes (or oats) and salt.

Put the dates in a small pan with 6 tablespoons of water and cook, covered, over a low heat for 5–8 minutes until softened, adding a splash more water if needed. Remove from the heat and mash the dates to a purée with the back of a fork, then stir in the peanut butter. Add the date mixture to the bowl and mix well until combined.

Spoon the date mixture into the prepared pan and spread it out into an even layer, pressing down firmly with the back of a wet spoon.

Bake for 20–25 minutes until firmed up and light golden around the edges; it will crisp up further when cool. Leave to cool completely in the pan, then lift out, using the baking parchment to help you, and cut into 16 bars. Store in an airtight container for 3–5 days.

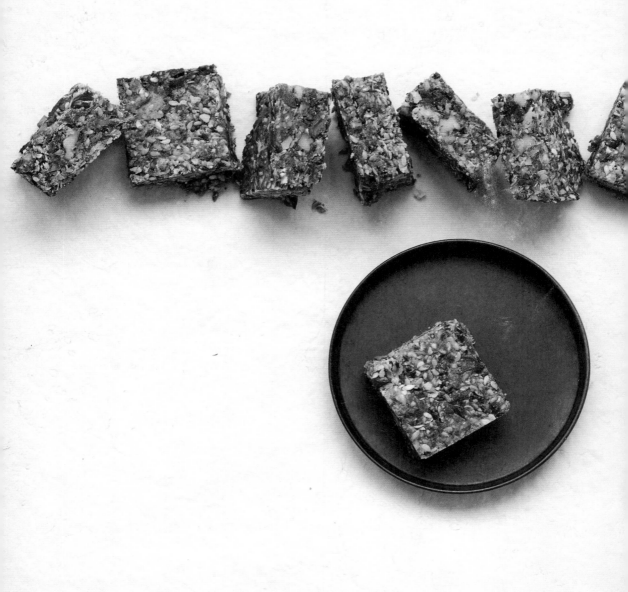

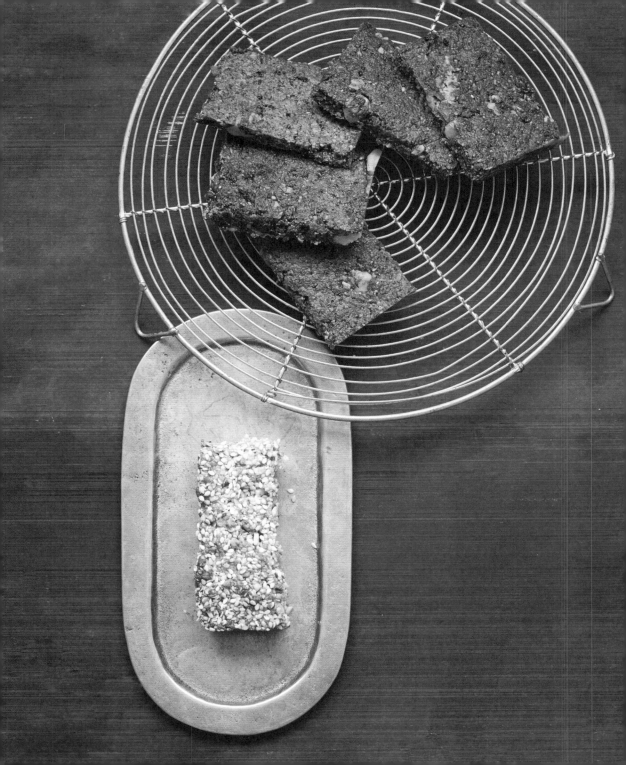

4 O'CLOCK BARS

Perfect if you are flagging mid-afternoon.

100 g/3½ oz. (dark) raisins
50 g/1¾ oz. soft dried apricots, roughly chopped
100 g/3½ oz. walnut pieces
100 g/3½ oz. sunflower seeds
75 g/2¾ oz. peanut butter (smooth or crunchy)
3 tablespoons good-quality honey
1 tablespoon chia seeds
50 g/1¾ oz. ground flaxseeds/linseeds

25 x 20-cm/10 x 8-inch baking pan, lined with baking parchment

MAKES 10

Preheat the oven to 180°C (350°F) Gas 4.

Put the raisins, apricots and 3 tablespoons of water in a small pan. Cover and cook over a medium-low heat for 5 minutes until soft.

Process half of the walnuts and sunflower seeds in a food processor for 2 minutes until very fine. Add the cooked dried fruit and any water in the pan, the peanut butter and honey, and process to a thick, coarse paste. Stir in the chia seeds, flaxseeds/linseeds and the reserved walnuts and sunflower seeds.

Spread the fruit and nut mixture evenly in the prepared pan. Bake for 20 minutes until firmed up and starting to turn golden around the edges. Mark into 10 bars then leave to sit for 10 minutes. When cooled slightly, turn out onto a wire rack to cool completely.

SESAME & TAHINI BARS

Protein-rich tahini is packed with minerals, numerous B vitamins as well as vitamin E.

125 g/4½ oz. good-quality honey
100 g/3½ oz. almond butter
6 tablespoons tahini
150 g/5½ oz. sesame seeds
150 g/5½ oz. almonds, roughly chopped
100 g/3½ oz. shelled unsalted pistachios, roughly chopped
60 g/2¼ oz. buckwheat flakes or quinoa flakes
¼ teaspoon sea salt

20-cm/8-inch baking pan, lined with baking parchment

MAKES 12

Preheat the oven to 180°C (350°F) Gas 4.

Gently melt the honey over a low heat. Remove from the heat and leave to cool slightly before stirring in the almond butter and tahini.

Meanwhile, mix together the sesame seeds, almonds, pistachios, buckwheat flakes (or quinoa flakes) and salt in a bowl. Pour in the honey mixture and stir to combine.

Tip the mixture into the prepared baking pan and press down into a firm even layer with the back of a wet spoon. Bake for 20 minutes until golden and firm. Mark into 12 bars and leave in the pan for 10 minutes before lifting out, using the baking parchment to help you. Separate into bars and leave to cool completely on a wire rack.

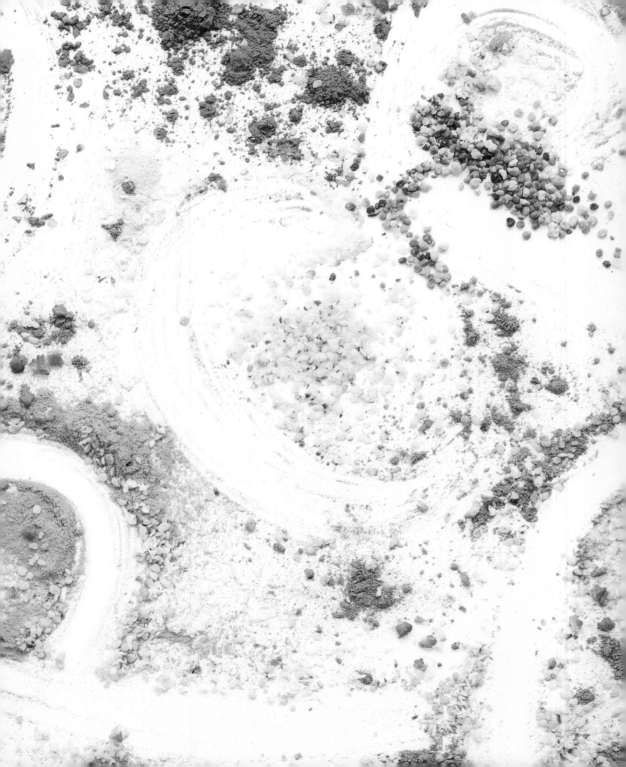

3

SUPERFOOD
SAVOURY

RAW
FALAFEL

A perfect post-exercise snack for when you fancy something savoury, rather than sweet. These also work well as a healthy addition to a lunchbox when served with humous.

85 g/3 oz. pumpkin seeds
55 g/2 oz. walnut pieces
3 sun-dried tomatoes in oil,
  drained and halved
a handful of flat leaf parsley,
  leaves and stalks
½ teaspoon dried oregano
1 garlic clove, peeled
1 tablespoon freshly squeezed
  lemon juice
2 teaspoons finely grated unwaxed
  lemon zest
3 tablespoons nutritional yeast
  flakes, plus extra 4 tablespoons
  for coating
sea salt and freshly ground
  black pepper

TO SERVE (OPTIONAL)
Little Gem lettuce leaves
humous
chopped fresh chilli/chile

MAKES 10

Put the pumpkin seeds and walnuts in a food processor and process for 2 minutes until very finely chopped and they start to form a coarse paste.

Add the sun-dried tomatoes, parsley, oregano, garlic and lemon juice to the food processor and blitz to a thick paste. Add the lemon zest and nutritional yeast flakes. Season with salt and pepper and stir until combined.

Put the nutritional yeast flakes for coating on a plate.

With damp hands, form the mixture into 10 large marble-sized balls, then roll each one in the extra nutritional yeast flakes until coated all over. Chill for 30 minutes to firm up and then serve or store in the fridge in an airtight container for up to 5 days.

Serve on their own or with Little Gem lettuce leaves, humous and chopped chilli/chile if you like.

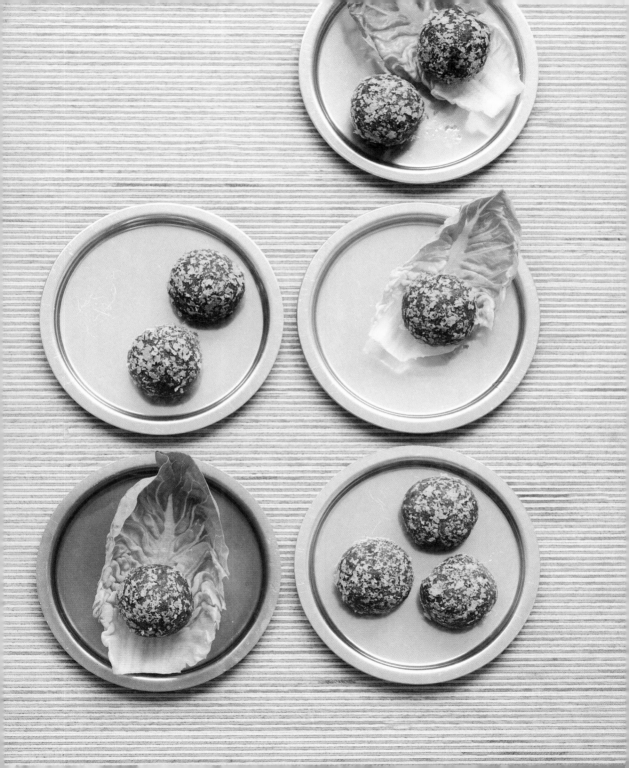

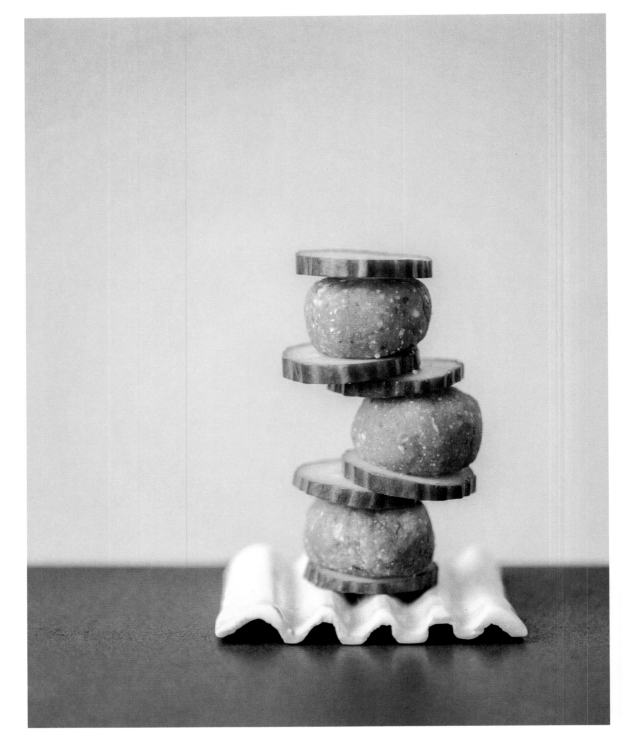

SUPER SNACKS

Miso and ginger give these nutty balls a health boost, as well as a burst of flavour. Ginger is a great stomach settler so if you're feeling nauseous or suffering from loss of appetite, then these balls could offer you a much-needed energy lift. The balls are each served between two slices of cucumber, which give a lovely, crisp freshness.

50 g/1¾ oz. cashew nuts
50 g/1¾ oz. sunflower seeds
40 g/1½ oz. quinoa flakes or jumbo rolled oats
2 soft dried pitted dates, chopped
2 teaspoons brown miso paste
1 tablespoon finely grated fresh root ginger
60 g/2¼ oz. peanut butter
1 tablespoon freshly squeezed lemon juice
15-cm/6-inch piece cucumber, cut into 24 thin slices, each about 3 mm/⅛ inch thick

MAKES 12

Blitz the cashews and sunflower seeds in a food processor until finely chopped. Add the rest of the ingredients, except the cucumber, and blend to a thick, coarse paste, occasionally scraping down the mixture from the sides when needed.

With damp hands, shape the cashew mixture into 12 walnut-sized balls and then flatten each one into a disc about 2 cm/¾ inch thick. Chill for 30 minutes to firm up.

Just before serving, place a snack ball between two slices of cucumber to make a type of cucumber 'sandwich'. Eat straightaway or store the balls (without the cucumber) in the fridge in an airtight container for up to 2 weeks. Place between the cucumber slices just before serving.

BEETROOT & GINGER BALLS

Beetroot provides iron, folic acid, magnesium and nitrates that can help to reduce blood pressure.

70 g/2½ oz. peeled raw beetroot/beet, chopped
70 g/2½ oz. sprouted chickpeas
2 tablespoons pumpkin seeds, roughly chopped, plus extra for topping
4-cm/1½-inch piece of fresh root ginger, peeled and grated
2 soft dried pitted dates, chopped
50 g/1¾ oz. cooked quinoa
3 tablespoons ground almonds
2 teaspoons acai powder (optional)

MAKES 10

Put the beetroot/beet, sprouted chickpeas and half of the pumpkin seeds in a food processor and process until very finely chopped. Add the ginger and dates, and process again to a thick, smooth-ish paste, occasionally scraping down the mixture from the sides when needed.

Put the cooked quinoa in a mixing bowl and mash roughly with the back of a fork to break down the grains, then add the beetroot/beet mixture, the rest of the pumpkin seeds, the ground almonds and acai powder, if using.

With damp hands, shape the beetroot/beet mixture into 10 walnut-sized balls and top each with a pumpkin seed, if you like. Chill for 30 minutes to firm up. Store in the fridge in an airtight container for up to 5 days.

LUNCHBOX PROTEIN BALLS

A great nutritious and protein-rich addition to a lunchbox, these balls can be served plain or stuffed into a flatbread.

70 g/2½ oz. sprouted lentils or chickpeas
50 g/1¾ oz. walnuts, roughly chopped
1 tablespoon toasted sesame seeds
1 garlic clove, crushed
1 teaspoon finely grated unwaxed lemon zest
2 teaspoons freshly squeezed lemon juice, plus extra, if needed
1 heaped teaspoon harissa paste
large pinch of sea salt
½ teaspoon red pepper flakes or ¼ teaspoon dried chilli flakes/hot red pepper flakes, plus extra for sprinkling (optional)

MAKES 8

Blitz the sprouted lentils (or chickpeas) and half of the walnuts in a food processor until very finely chopped. Scrape the mixture into a mixing bowl and stir in the remaining walnuts and the rest of the ingredients.

With damp hands, shape the walnut mixture into 8 walnut-sized balls and sprinkle a little extra red pepper flakes or chilli flakes/hot red pepper flakes over the top of each one, if you like. Chill for 30 minutes to firm up and then serve or store in the fridge in an airtight container for up to 2 weeks.

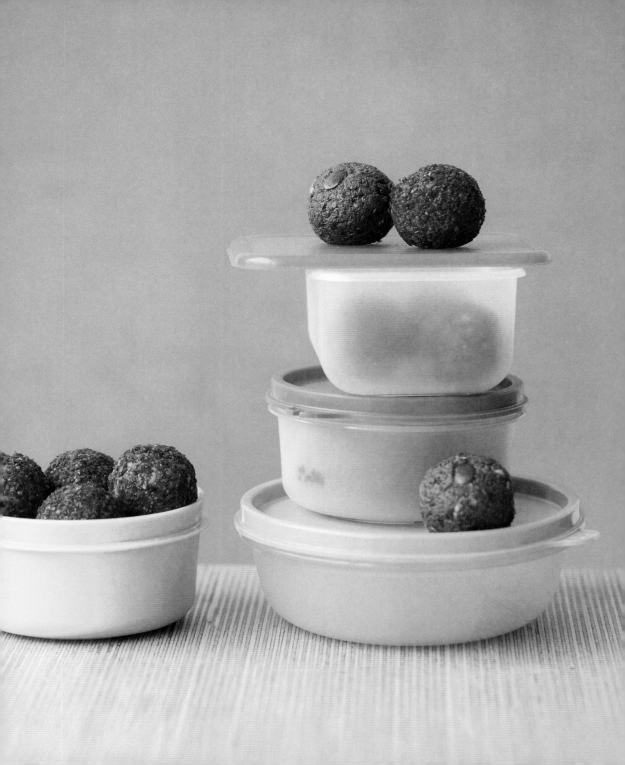

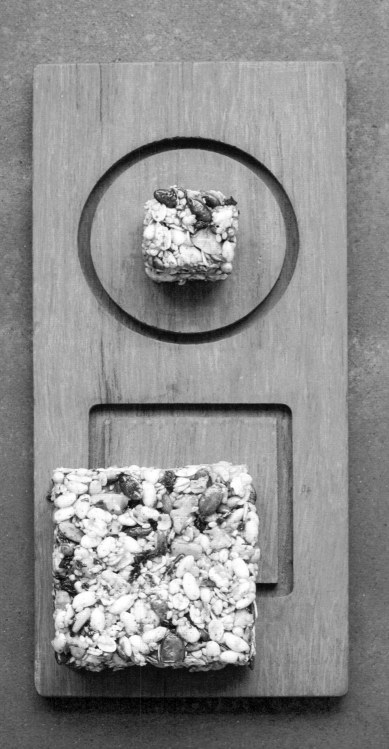

SAVOURY GRANOLA BARS

These energy-fuelled bars hold together well, meaning they are easily transportable – perfect for eating while out and about. Don't be put off by the list of ingredients, they are easy to make and require no baking. You could use shop-bought kale chips or follow the recipe for Kale Chips with Dukkah (see page 104), but leave out the dukkah.

60 g/2¼ oz. walnuts
55 g/2 oz. pumpkin seeds
55 g/2 oz. sesame seeds
90 g/3¼ oz. jumbo rolled oats
40 g/1½ oz. wholegrain unsweetened puffed rice
10 g/¼ oz. Kale Chips (see page 104, or use shop-bought), torn into small pieces
1 teaspoon hot smoked paprika
2 tablespoons coconut oil
175 g/6 oz. brown rice syrup
3 tablespoons almond butter
sea salt, to taste

25 x 20-cm/10 x 8-inch baking pan, lined with clingfilm/plastic wrap, leaving enough overhang to fold over the top

MAKES 15

Put the walnuts in a large, dry frying pan/skillet and toast for 5 minutes over a medium-low heat, tossing the pan occasionally, until the nuts start to colour. Remove from the pan and roughly chop. Place in a mixing bowl.

Toast the pumpkin seeds in the pan for 3 minutes, tossing occasionally, until starting to colour, then remove. Repeat with the sesame seeds. Place the seeds in the bowl with the walnuts and stir in the oats, puffed rice, kale chips and smoked paprika. Season with a little salt to taste, and stir well until everything is combined.

Gently heat the coconut oil and rice syrup in a pan until melted. Remove from the heat and stir in the almond butter. Pour into the dry ingredients and mix well.

Tip the puffed rice mixture into the prepared baking pan and spread out into an even layer with the back of a wet spoon, pressing it down firmly. Fold over the clingfilm/plastic wrap to cover the top of the mixture, then chill for 1 hour to firm up. Cut into 15 bars. Keep stored in the fridge in an airtight container for up to 1 week.

CAULI-CHICKPEA POWER BALLS

These are a twist on classic falafel with the addition of cauliflower and chia seeds. Baked in the oven, rather than fried, the balls can be served warm or cold as a nutritious snack, or as a filling for a wholegrain pitta or tortilla wrap with tahini, salad leaves and a hit of chilli sauce. Gluten-free gram flour is made from ground chickpeas and lends a golden colour and protein-boost to the balls.

400-g/14-oz. can chickpeas, rinsed, drained well and patted dry
250 g/9 oz. cauliflower florets
3 spring onions/scallions, roughly chopped
2 garlic cloves, peeled
2 teaspoons ground coriander
1 teaspoon ground cumin
2 rounded tablespoons gram flour
2 tablespoons chia seeds
1 teaspoon baking powder
finely grated zest of 1 unwaxed lemon
40 g/1½ oz. sesame seeds
sea salt and freshly ground black pepper
cold-pressed rapeseed oil, for brushing

baking sheet, lightly greased with cold-pressed rapeseed oil

MAKES 16

Put the chickpeas, cauliflower, spring onions/scallions and garlic in a food processor and process to a coarse paste. Stir in the spices, gram flour, chia seeds, baking powder and lemon zest. Season with salt and pepper to taste and stir well until combined.

Put the sesame seeds on a plate.

With damp hands, form the chickpea mixture into 16 large, walnut-sized balls, then roll each one in the sesame seeds until coated all over. Chill for 30 minutes to firm up.

Preheat the oven to 190°C (375°F) Gas 5. Place the balls on the greased baking sheet, brush them lightly with oil and cook in the oven for 30–35 minutes, turning once, until golden and crisp. Eat warm or leave to cool and store in the fridge in an airtight container for 3–5 days.

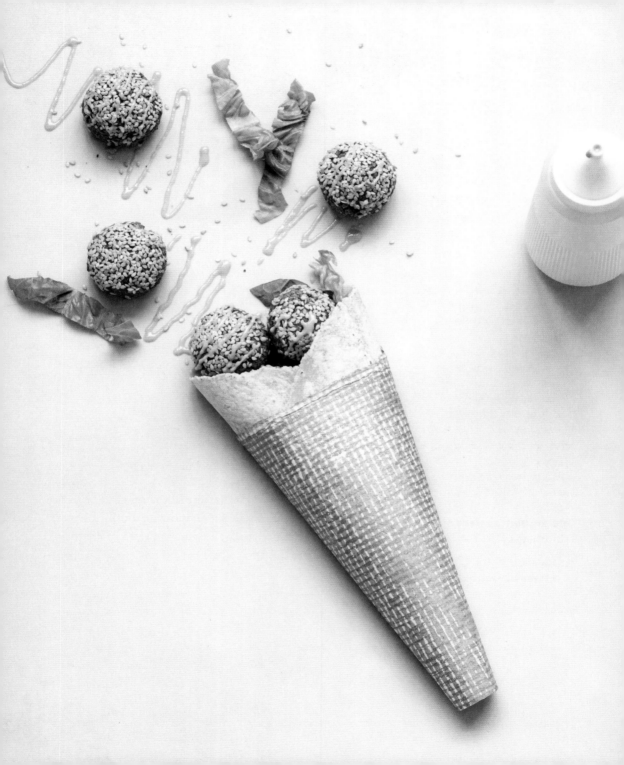

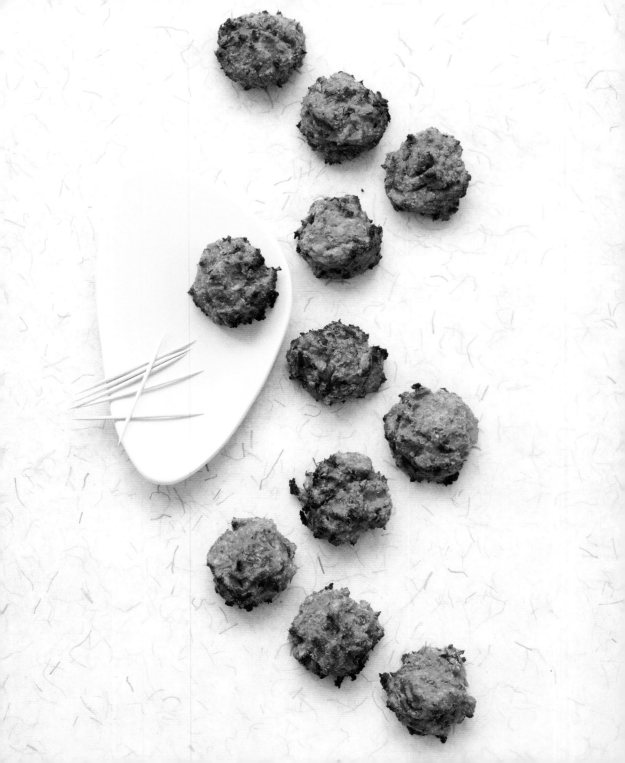

SWEET POTATO & QUINOA BITES

The combination of ras el hanout, ginger and coriander/cilantro gives these crispy morsels a Moroccan feel. Ginger is a great asset in the superfood kitchen, giving a warming, zingy lift to food, as well as being an effective digestive aid, anti-inflammatory and analgesic for joints.

400 g/14 oz. sweet potato, peeled and cut into large chunks
70 g/2½ oz. cooked quinoa
2.5-cm/1-inch piece of fresh root ginger, grated (no need to peel)
2 large garlic cloves, finely chopped
a handful of chopped coriander/cilantro leaves
2 teaspoons ras el hanout
3 tablespoons almond flour
1 egg, lightly beaten
sea salt and freshly ground black pepper
cold-pressed rapeseed oil, for brushing

2 baking sheets, lined with baking parchment and lightly greased with cold-pressed rapeseed oil

MAKES 20

Steam the sweet potato for 10–15 minutes until tender. Leave to cool slightly, then coarsely grate the sweet potato into a mixing bowl. Add the cooked quinoa to the bowl and roughly mash with the back of a fork to break the grains down slightly. Stir in the ginger, garlic, coriander/cilantro leaves, ras el hanout and almond flour. Season the mixture with salt and pepper, then stir in the egg until everything is combined.

Rather than rolling the mixture into balls in your hands, use a tablespoon as a mould – take heaped tablespoonfuls of the sweet potato mixture and 'plop' them out in mounds onto the prepared baking sheets. Chill them for 30 minutes to firm up.

Meanwhile, preheat the oven to 190°C (375°F) Gas 5.

Brush the tops of the bites with cold-pressed rapeseed oil and bake for 25–30 minutes until crisp on the outside and light golden. Eat warm or cold. Store in the fridge in an airtight container for 3–5 days.

JAPANESE
RICE BALLS

Nutritionally, brown rice is superior to white rice and is a good source of fibre – it also has a lovely nutty flavour. To make these Japanese rice balls, or onigiri, use short-grain rice, rather than long-grain or basmati, as its sticky texture will ensure the balls hold together.

175 g/6 oz. short-grain brown rice, rinsed well
2 teaspoons black sesame seeds
2 teaspoons hulled hemp seeds
¼ teaspoon togarashi spice mix, plus extra for sprinkling (optional)
½ sheet toasted nori, cut into 10 strips, each about 4 x 1 cm/ 1½ x ½ inch in size
sea salt, to taste

FILLINGS (OPTIONAL)
Japanese pickles, cut into small pieces
kimchi, finely chopped
smoked tofu, cut into small cubes
grated cooked egg yolk

MAKES 10

Put the rice in a pan. Pour over 275 ml/generous 1 cup cold water (it should cover the rice by about 1 cm/½ inch) and bring to the boil. Cover the pan with a lid, turn the heat to its lowest setting, and cook for 20–25 minutes until the rice is tender and all the water has been absorbed. Turn off the heat and leave to stand for 15 minutes.

Mix together the black sesame seeds, hemp seeds and togarashi, then stir the mixture into the rice.

To make plain onigiri, take a small piece of clingfilm/ plastic wrap in the palm of one hand and place 2 tablespoons of rice in the centre. Gather up the edges of the clingfilm/plastic wrap and twist the top, then gently press the rice into a triangle, ball or cylindrical shape.

To make filled onigiri, follow the instructions above. Put the rice in the centre of the clingfilm/plastic wrap and press it into a disc with wet fingers. Place a piece of pickle, kimchi, smoked tofu or ½ teaspoon of egg yolk in the centre and shape the rice around, using the clingfilm/ plastic wrap to help, to encase the filling. Next, shape the rice into a triangle or ball shape.

Remove the clingfilm/plastic wrap and stick a strip of nori around the base, then finish with a sprinkling of togarashi on top, if liked. Eat straightaway or store, covered, in the fridge for up to 2 days.

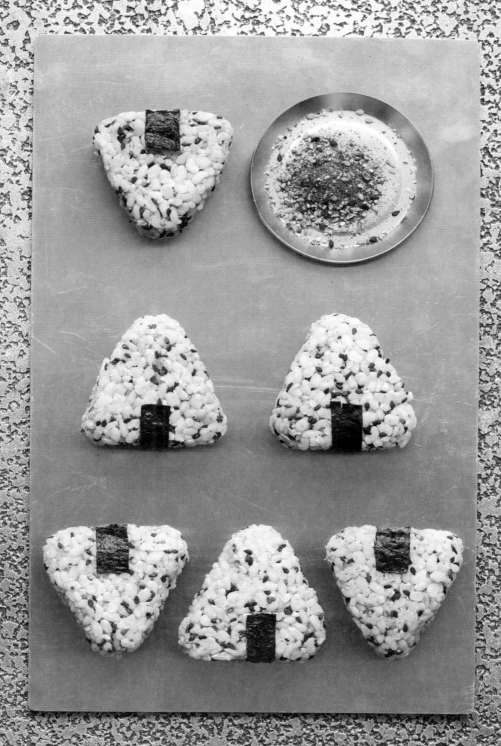

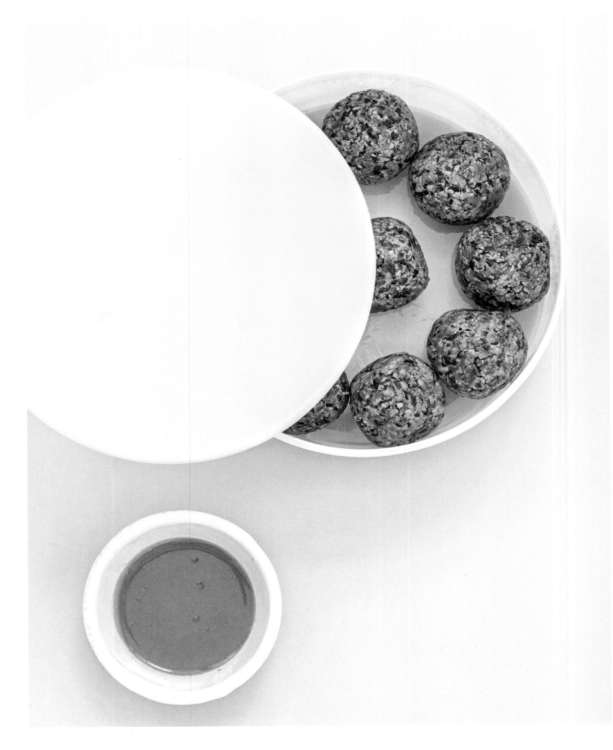

TOFU, GINGER & CHILLI/CHILI BALLS

Light in flavour but not in nutritional value, these tofu balls benefit from the addition of chilli flakes/hot red pepper flakes, spring onions/scallions, garlic, ginger, turmeric and coriander/cilantro leaves. Protein, iron, calcium, magnesium, zinc, selenium, copper and vitamin B1 are all found in beneficial amounts. Serve the balls plain or with a sweet chilli/chili dipping sauce.

225 g/8 oz. tofu, drained well
2.5-cm/1-inch piece of fresh root ginger, peeled and finely grated
1 teaspoon dried chilli flakes/hot red pepper flakes
2 garlic cloves, grated
2 large spring onions/scallions, very finely chopped
1 teaspoon ground turmeric
a handful of chopped coriander/cilantro leaves
½ teaspoon sea salt
1 tablespoon dried nori flakes
2 tablespoons cornflour/cornstarch
cold-pressed rapeseed oil, for frying

MAKES 12

Wrap the tofu in paper towels and press firmly to remove as much water as possible. Coarsely grate the tofu and squeeze out any surplus water still in the tofu.

Put the grated tofu in a mixing bowl with the ginger, chilli flakes/hot red pepper flakes, garlic, spring onions/scallions, turmeric, coriander/cilantro, salt and nori flakes. Mix well, then sprinkle over the cornflour/cornstarch and stir until combined.

With damp hands, shape the mixture into 12 walnut-sized balls and place in the fridge for 30 minutes to firm up or until ready to cook.

Heat a generous amount of rapeseed oil in a large frying pan/skillet and cook the balls in batches of four for 8–10 minutes, turning them occasionally until golden all over. Drain on paper towels and serve warm or at room temperature. The balls can be left to cool and then stored in the fridge in an airtight container for up to 3 days.

DUKKAH BEAN BALLS

These kidney bean balls are flavoured with dukkah, the Egyptian fragrant spice, nut and seed mix with a hint of chilli/chile. A take on falafel, they can be eaten as a snack on their own or dunked into humous, guacamole or a mint yogurt dip. Alternatively, stuff them into a wrap, taco shell or pitta bread with lots of salad for a full meal.

1 small onion, chopped
2 garlic cloves, peeled
400-g/14-oz. can red kidney beans, drained and rinsed
40 g/1½ oz. carrot, finely grated
2 teaspoons gram flour
2 tablespoons Dukkah (see page 104)
sea salt and freshly ground black pepper
olive oil, for brushing

baking sheet, lined with baking parchment

MAKES 10

Put the onion and garlic in a food processor and blitz to a coarse paste. Add the kidney beans and process again to make a coarse purée (you want to retain some chunks of kidney bean), occasionally scraping the mixture down the sides when needed. Stir in the carrot, gram flour and dukkah, then season with salt and pepper.

With damp hands, form the mixture into 10 walnut-sized balls, place on the prepared baking sheet and chill for 30 minutes to firm up.

Meanwhile, preheat the oven to 190°C (375°F) Gas 5.

Generously brush the balls with olive oil and bake in the oven for 25 minutes, turning occasionally, or until golden brown all over. Eat warm or cold. The balls will keep stored in the fridge in an airtight container for up to 3 days.

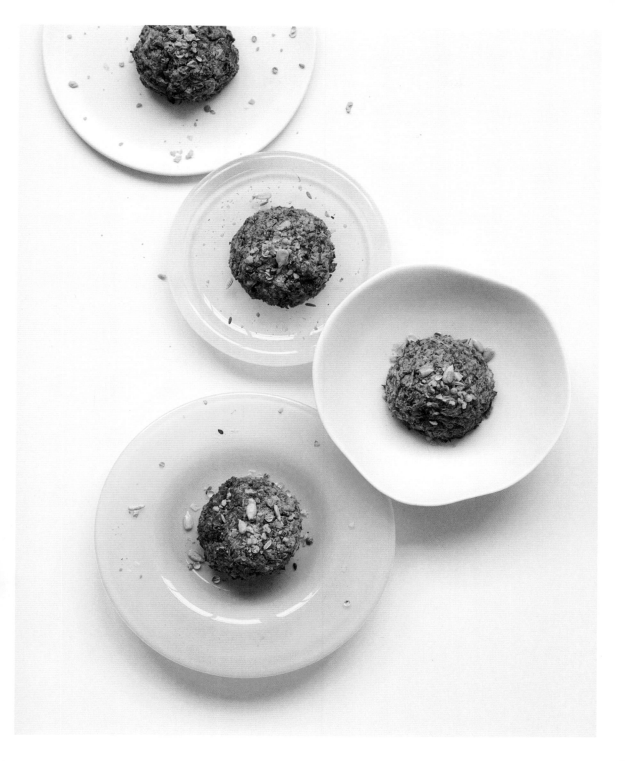

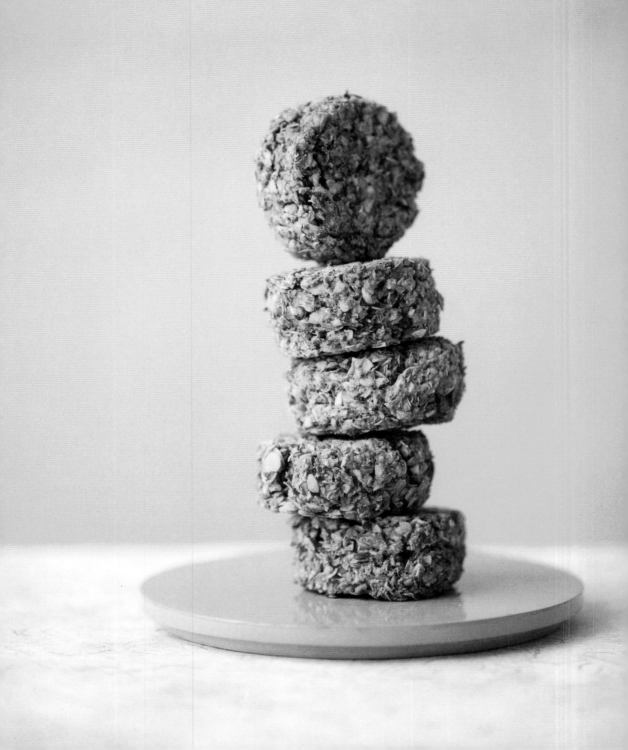

POWER GREEN BEAN BALLS

Like other pulses, broad (fava) beans are naturally low in fat and high in protein and fibre. They're also rich in folate, B vitamins, iron, magnesium and zinc – perfect for providing sustained amounts of energy. You need to plan ahead when making these bean balls, as the broad/fava beans require pre-soaking. However, unlike other beans, they don't require pre-cooking. Delicious with a minty yogurt dip.

200 g/7 oz. dried split broad/fava beans, soaked overnight
5 spring onions/scallions, roughly chopped
3 garlic cloves, peeled
2 tablespoons pumpkin seeds
a handful of coriander/cilantro leaves
a handful of parsley leaves
1 teaspoon ground cumin
1 teaspoon ground coriander
1 teaspoon baking powder
3 tablespoons gram flour
sea salt and freshly ground black pepper
olive oil, for brushing

baking sheet, lined with baking parchment

MAKES 16

Preheat the oven to 180°C (350°F) Gas 4.

Drain the soaked beans and put them in a food processor with the spring onions/scallions, garlic, pumpkin seeds and herbs. Process to a coarse paste, occasionally scraping down the mixture from the sides when needed.

Add the spices, baking powder and gram flour. Season with salt and pepper to taste and stir to make a coarse paste – it will be slightly wet but will hold together when cooked.

With damp hands, form the mixture into 16 large, walnut-sized balls and put them on the prepared baking sheet. Flatten the tops slightly, brush each one with a little olive oil, then bake for 20–25 minutes, turning once, until firm and golden in places. Serve warm or leave to cool. Store in the fridge in an airtight container for 3–5 days.

SATAY RICE BALLS

These delicious morsels capture the flavours of classic satay in a rice ball. Brown rice is a must for its wide range of vitamins, minerals and fibre – white just doesn't cut it. There are a number of ways to serve the balls, either pre- or post-baking, on their own, or with a garlicky roasted red (bell) pepper dip.

125 g/4½ oz. brown basmati rice
10 g/¼ oz. desiccated/dried unsweetened shredded coconut
2 spring onions/scallions, roughly chopped
60 g/2¼ oz. peanut butter (crunchy or smooth)
2.5-cm/1-inch piece of fresh root ginger, peeled and roughly chopped
2 garlic cloves, peeled
2 teaspoons tamari or light soy sauce
½ teaspoon dried chilli flakes/hot red pepper flakes
1 teaspoon ground turmeric
a handful of coriander/cilantro, leaves and stalks
1 teaspoon coconut oil, plus extra for cooking
40 g/1½ oz. sesame seeds
2 tablespoons dried nori flakes
sea salt and freshly ground black pepper

MAKES 13

Put the rice in a pan, cover with plenty of cold water and bring to the boil. Turn the heat down to its lowest setting and simmer, covered with a lid, for 25 minutes, or until cooked.

While the rice is cooking, toast the coconut in a small, dry frying pan/skillet, tossing the pan regularly until it starts to turn light golden; take care as it can easily burn. Remove from the heat and tip the coconut into a food processor with the spring onions/scallions, peanut butter, ginger, garlic, tamari (or soy sauce), chilli flakes/hot red pepper flakes, turmeric, coriander/cilantro and coconut oil.

When the rice is ready, drain it if necessary, then tip half of the rice into the food processor. Process until the mixture forms a coarse paste. Stir in the rest of the rice and season with salt and pepper.

Mix together the sesame seeds and nori flakes on a plate.

With damp hands, form the rice mixture into 13 large, walnut-sized balls, then roll in the sesame seed mixture until coated all over. The balls can be served at this point while still warm or left to cool. Store in the fridge in an airtight container for 3–5 days.

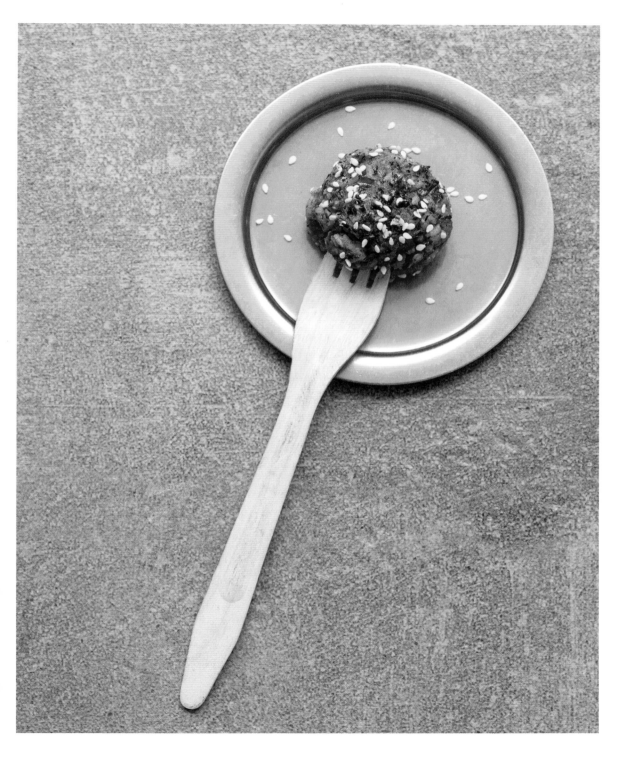

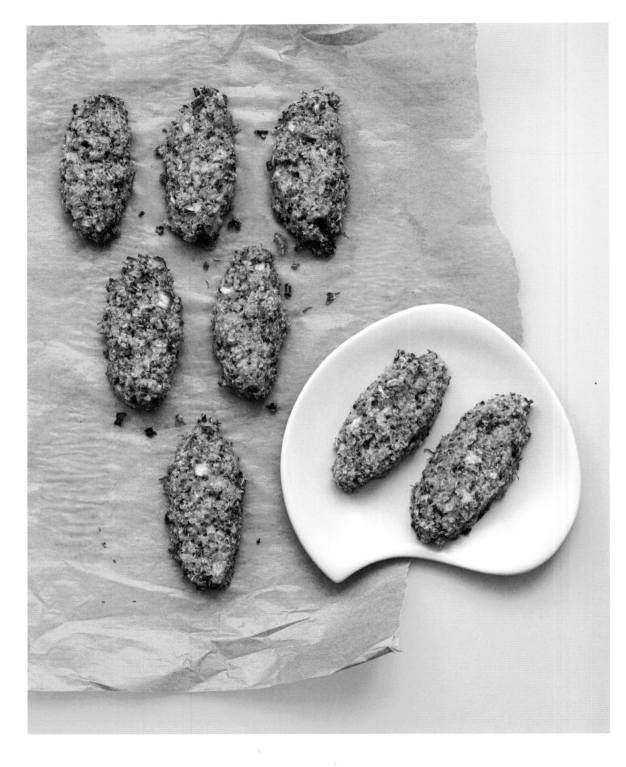

QUINOA, ALMOND & BROCCOLI BITES

These tasty, savoury morsels are easy to prepare and make a nutritious, fibre-rich and protein-fuelled snack or addition to a lunchbox. If cooking the quinoa from scratch, you'll need about 40 g/1½ oz. of the uncooked grains.

175 g/6 oz. broccoli florets
2 spring onions/scallions, finely chopped
115 g/4 oz. cooked quinoa
50 g/1¾ oz. Cheddar cheese, grated
2 tablespoons ground almonds
1 UK large/US extra-large egg, lightly beaten
sea salt and freshly ground black pepper

baking sheet, lined with baking parchment

MAKES 10–12

Preheat the oven to 200°C (400°F) Gas 6.

Blitz the broccoli in a food processor until very finely chopped, and scrape it into a bowl. Stir in the spring onions/scallions, cooked quinoa, Cheddar, ground almonds and egg. Season well with salt and pepper, and stir until combined.

Form the broccoli mixture into 10–12 sausage-shaped patties, each about 5 cm/2 inches long (the mixture is fairly wet, but will hold together when pressed). Place the 'bites' on the prepared baking sheet and cook in the oven for 25 minutes or until firmed up and golden in places. The bites can be eaten warm or cold and will keep in the fridge in an airtight container for up to 3 days.

4

SUPERFOOD
SNACKS

CASHEW 'CHEESE' BALLS

Cashews make a remarkably good vegan alternative to soft cheese – simply soak and blend them with a splash of water until smooth and creamy, then form into balls or pot into ramekins. Healthwise, not only do cashews have a lower fat content than most other nuts, much of it is unsaturated and the heart-friendly monounsaturated type.

125 g/4½ oz. cashew nuts
½ teaspoon sea salt
1 garlic clove, crushed
2 teaspoons freshly squeezed lemon juice
4 tablespoons nutritional yeast flakes
freshly ground black pepper, to taste

TO COAT, CHOOSE FROM
toasted walnuts or shelled unsalted pistachios, finely chopped
mixed freshly chopped herbs, such as oregano, chives and parsley
ground almonds mixed with nutritional yeast flakes
Dukkah (see page 104)

MAKES 10

Put the cashews in a bowl, cover with warm water and leave to soak for 2 hours until softened. Drain the cashews and tip them into a food processor or heavy-duty blender.

Pour 3 tablespoons of water into the processor or blender and add the salt, garlic, lemon juice and nutritional yeast flakes. Blend to a thick, smooth-ish purée, occasionally scraping down the mixture from the sides when needed. Season with pepper, then chill the cashew mixture for 30 minutes to firm up slightly.

Shape the mixture into 10 walnut-sized balls and then roll them in the coating(s) of your choice. They will keep in the fridge in an airtight container for up to 3 days.

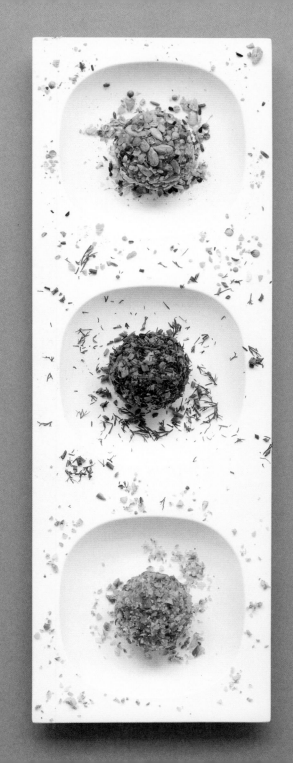

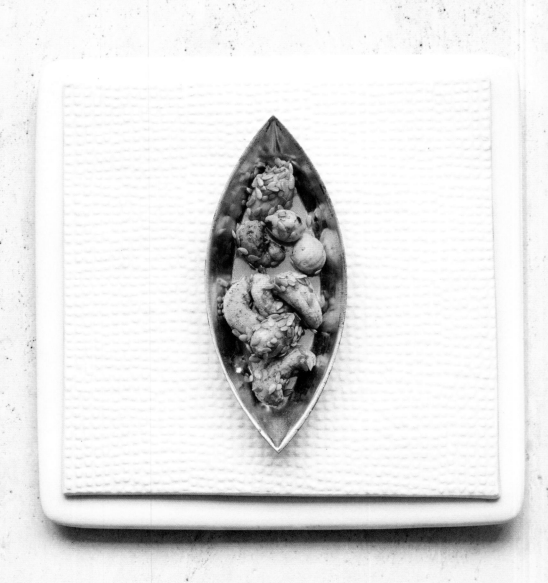

HONEY-SPICE NUT CLUSTERS

A small handful of these sticky, cinnamon-spiced nuts makes an easy and convenient snack when energy levels are flagging. Naturally sweet, cinnamon is said to have a regulatory effect on blood sugar levels and may help to reduce inflammation in the body.

100 g/3½ oz. mixed nuts, such as cashews, almonds and hazelnuts
2 teaspoons good-quality honey
½ teaspoon coconut oil
½ teaspoon ground cinnamon
pinch of sea salt
2 teaspoons flaxseeds/linseeds
1 teaspoon sesame seeds

baking sheet, lined with baking parchment

MAKES 100 G/3½ OZ.

Preheat the oven to 160°C (325°F) Gas 3.

Spread the nuts out on the lined baking sheet and toast in the oven for 8 minutes, turning once, until they start to turn light golden.

Meanwhile, gently heat the honey and coconut oil in a small pan until melted, then stir in the cinnamon and salt. (If the weather is warm it may be enough to just mix everything together without heating.)

Remove the baking sheet from the oven, transfer the toasted nuts to the pan and turn until coated in the honey mixture. Return the nuts to the lined baking sheet and bake in the oven for 5 minutes, or until golden, turning once so they cook evenly.

Scatter the flaxseeds/linseeds and sesame seeds over the nuts and turn so that everything sticks together in small clusters. Leave to cool on the baking sheet. Eat at once or keep in an airtight container for up to 3 days.

SEAWEED & SESAME CASHEWS

These tamari-coated cashews are given a health boost with the addition of mineral-rich nori and sesame seeds, which are loaded with beneficial fats. Cashews provide a range of health benefits, and are a good source of copper. This plays a number of vital roles in the body from the development of bone and connective tissue to energy production, iron absorption and the elimination of free radicals.

100 g/3½ oz. cashew nuts
2 teaspoons tamari
1 teaspoon good-quality honey
1 teaspoon coconut oil
2 teaspoons sesame seeds
1 heaped teaspoon dried seaweed flakes, such as nori, dulse, smoked dulse or wakame
pinch of dried chilli flakes/hot red pepper flakes

baking sheet, lined with baking parchment

MAKES 100 G/3½ OZ.

Preheat the oven to 160°C (325°F) Gas 3.

Spread the cashews out on the lined baking sheet and toast in the oven for 8 minutes, turning once, until they start to turn light golden.

Meanwhile, gently heat the tamari, honey and coconut oil in a small pan until melted, then stir in the sesame seeds, seaweed flakes and chilli flakes/hot red pepper flakes. (If the weather is warm it may be enough to just mix everything together without heating.)

Remove the baking sheet from the oven, transfer the toasted cashews to the pan and turn until coated in the tamari mixture. Return the cashews to the lined baking sheet and bake in the oven for 5 minutes or until golden, turning once so they cook evenly.

Leave to cool on the baking sheet. Eat the cashews at once or keep in an airtight container for up to 3 days.

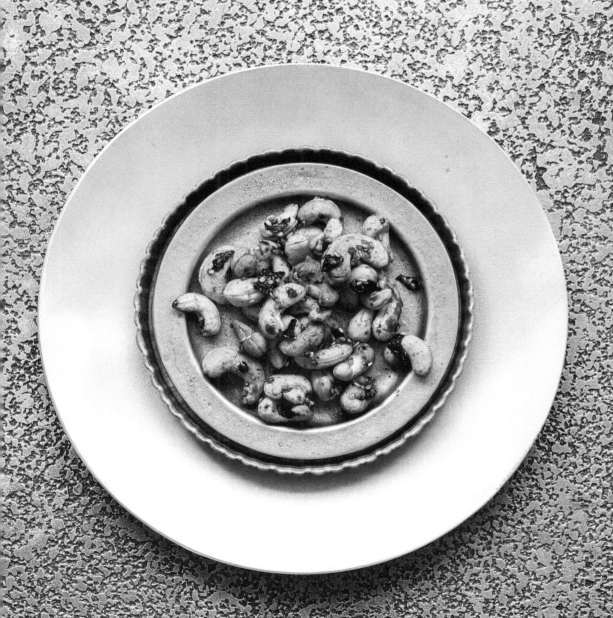

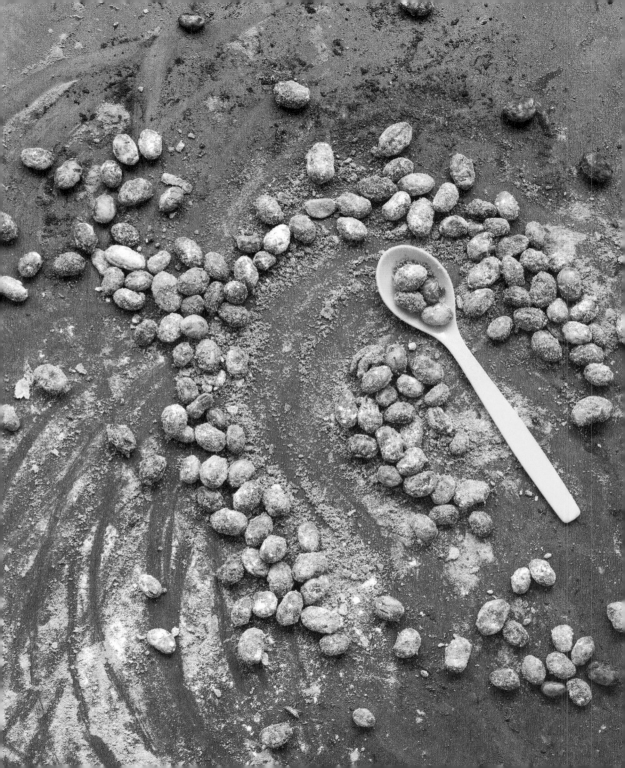

WASABI-ROASTED EDAMAME

Keeping a bag of edamame (young soya beans) in the freezer ensures you have a convenient snack-in-waiting. They can be transformed into falafel-type snack balls, puréed into vivid-green dips or coated in spices and roasted, as here. Edamame (young soya beans) are unusual in the plant world in that they are a complete protein, meaning they contain all nine essential amino acids. They're also brimming with minerals, such as iron, calcium, magnesium, potassium and zinc.

150 g/5½ oz. frozen edamame
    beans, defrosted
2 teaspoons cold-pressed
    rapeseed oil
1 teaspoon wasabi powder,
    or to taste
sea salt, to taste

*baking sheet, lined with baking
    parchment*

MAKES 150 G/5½ OZ.

Preheat the oven to 180°C (350°F) Gas 4.

Pat dry the edamame with paper towels and place on the prepared baking sheet. Pour the oil over the beans, toss with your hands until they are coated, then spread out on the baking sheet. Toast in the oven for 15 minutes, then remove and sprinkle the wasabi powder over them and season with salt. Turn the edamame until coated in the wasabi and return to the oven for another 15–20 minutes until crisp and golden.

Sprinkle over more wasabi or salt, to taste, if needed. Leave on the baking sheet to cool and crisp up further. Store in an airtight container for up to 3 days – they may lose their crispness slightly, but will still taste good.

VARIATION

Try experimenting with different types of beans and flavourings. Chickpeas are delicious and crisp up well in the oven to make a tasty snack. Simply rinse, drain and pat dry a 400-g/14-oz. can of chickpeas. Coat in 1 tablespoon olive oil and 2 teaspoons spice mix of your choice, and roast in the same way as the edamame, above.

BHEL PURI

A popular Indian street food snack, there are many versions of bhel puri, but it should always be a mixture of sour, hot, sweet and tangy flavours, and soft and crunchy textures. This version may not be completely authentic, but it captures the essence of the snack, although do feel free to swap the ingredients depending on what you have to hand. The traditional way to serve the snack is in a newspaper cone.

2 teaspoons coconut oil
40 g/1½ oz. shelled unsalted peanuts
2.5-cm/1-inch piece of fresh root ginger, grated (no need to peel)
25 g/1 oz. wholegrain unsweetened puffed rice
40 g/1½ oz. Crispy Chickpeas (see variation on page 99, optional)
½ teaspoon chaat masala spice mix
¼–½ medium-hot green chilli/chile, deseeded and diced
¼ small red onion, diced
1 teaspoon black sesame seeds
finely grated zest of 1 unwaxed lime
55 g/2 oz. fresh mango flesh, diced, or 2 vine-ripened tomatoes, deseeded and diced
sea salt, to taste

SERVES 2–3

Heat the coconut oil in a large frying pan/skillet over a medium heat, then add the peanuts and fry, stirring, for 2–3 minutes or until they start to smell toasted. Scoop out the nuts with a slotted spoon onto paper towels to drain and cool.

Turn down the heat slightly, add the ginger to the pan and cook for a minute or so until crisp, then drain and cool on paper towels.

Tip the cooled nuts and ginger into a mixing bowl and add the puffed rice, chickpeas (if using), chaat masala, chilli/chile, red onion, sesame seeds and lime zest. Season with salt to taste and stir until combined. Add the mango or tomatoes – it's best to do this just before serving so the puffed rice stays crisp. Serve in paper cones!

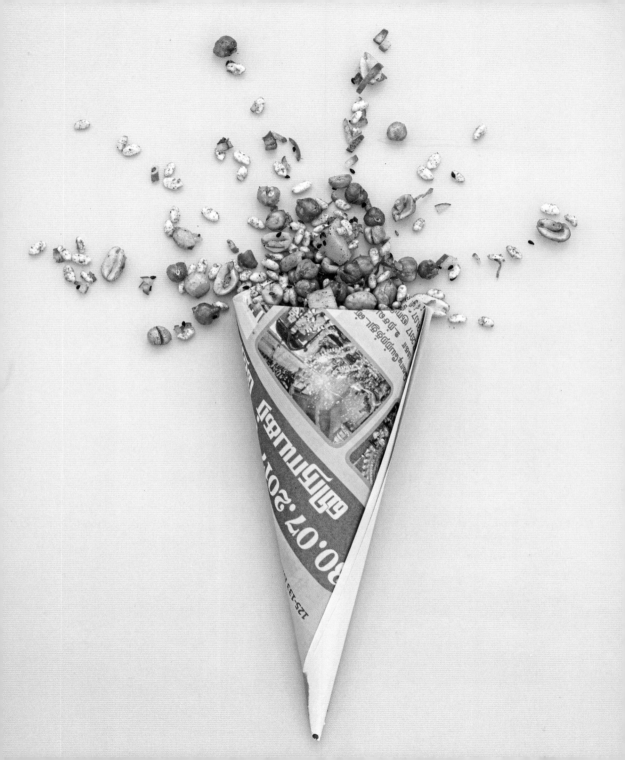

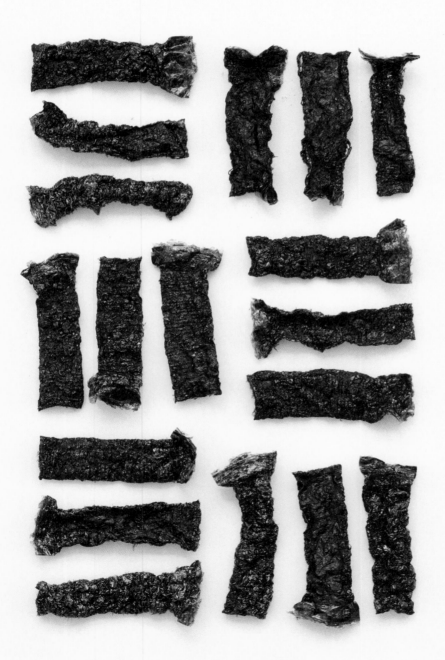

NORI MISO CRISPS

Very easy and very moreish… these crispy strips of nori are flavoured with brown miso and sprinkled with sesame seeds. You can also flavour them with wasabi paste and they are equally good.

2 teaspoons brown miso paste, or type of your choice
3 sheets toasted nori
½ teaspoon super-greens powder
½ teaspoon sesame seeds

baking sheet, lined with baking parchment

MAKES 24

Preheat the oven to 160°C (325°F) Gas 3.

Mix the miso paste with 2 teaspoons of water and brush it over one half of each sheet of nori. Sprinkle the super-greens powder and the sesame seeds over the miso-coated nori.

Fold the nori sheet in half to encase the filling and press down lightly so the two halves stick together.

Cut each sheet of nori into 8 strips, each 2 cm/¾ inch wide, and place on the prepared baking sheet. Cook in the oven for 5–7 minutes until crisp.

Leave to cool on the baking sheet, then eat straightaway or store in an airtight container for up to 1 day. They will keep for longer but tend to lose their crispness over time.

KALE CHIPS
WITH DUKKAH

I like to keep a jar of the Egyptian nut and seed mix, dukkah, to hand in the kitchen. It's perfect for adding a flavour boost to salads, dips, roasted vegetables, eggs and wraps, and can be used to make the Dukkah Bean Balls on page 82. Here, it's used as a flavouring and to give a nutrient-rich lift to kale chips.

70 g/2½ oz. kale, tough stalks removed, leaves torn into bite-sized pieces
1 teaspoon olive oil or coconut oil, melted

DUKKAH
50 g/1¾ oz. walnuts
40 g/1½ oz. hazelnuts
3 tablespoons coriander seeds
1 tablespoon cumin seeds
3 tablespoons sesame seeds
3 tablespoons pumpkin seeds
3 tablespoons sunflower seeds
½ teaspoon dried chilli flakes/hot red pepper flakes
sea salt, to taste

baking sheet, lined with baking parchment

MAKES 60 G/2¼ OZ.

Preheat the oven to 150°C (300°F) Gas 2.

For the dukkah, put the walnuts and hazelnuts on the lined baking sheet and toast in the oven for 10 minutes, turning once, until they start to colour. Tip into a bowl.

Meanwhile, put the coriander and cumin seeds in a large, dry frying pan/skillet and toast over a medium-low heat for 1–2 minutes, tossing occasionally, until they start to smell aromatic. Add to the bowl with the nuts.

Toast the sesame, pumpkin and sunflower seeds in the pan for 3–4 minutes, tossing occasionally, until the seeds start to colour. Add to the bowl. Stir in the chilli flakes/hot red pepper flakes, season with salt and leave to cool. When cool, transfer to a spice grinder or use a pestle and mortar to grind to a coarse, crumbly mixture.

Put the prepared kale in a bowl, add the oil and massage it into the leaves. Spread them out on the same lined baking sheet and toast for 15 minutes, turning once, until crisp – do not let the kale go brown as it can taste bitter.

Place the kale in a shallow bowl. Add 2 tablespoons of dukkah and mix to coat thoroughly with your hands. Eat at once or store in an airtight container for up to 1 day. They will keep for longer but tend to lose their crispness.

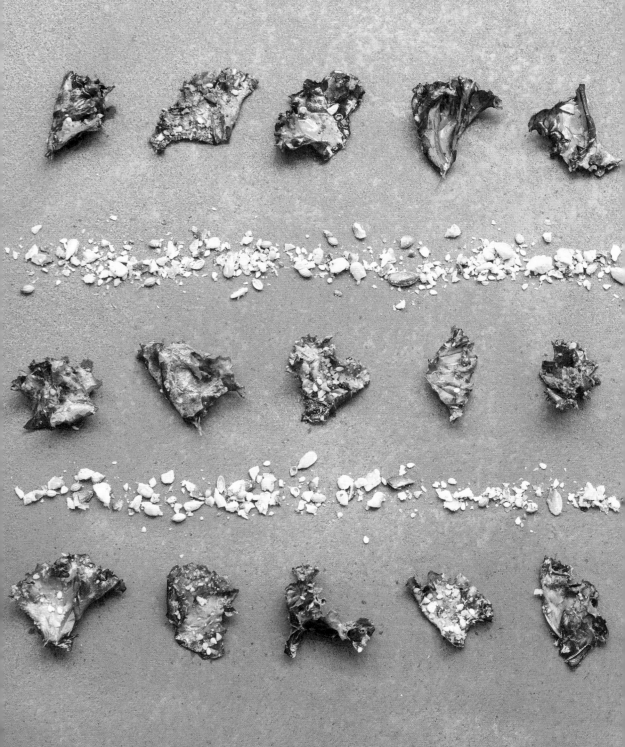

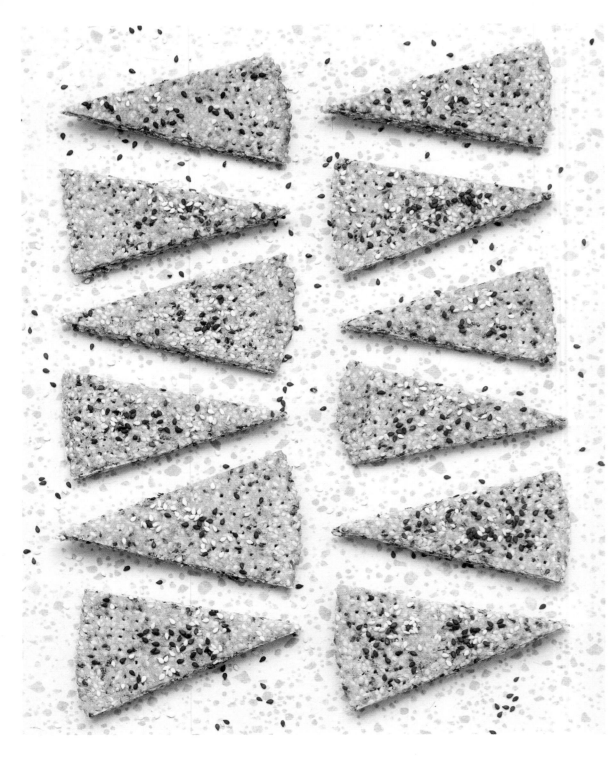

SESAME & NORI BUCKWHEAT CAKES

Despite its name, buckwheat is actually a seed rather than a grain and it is gluten-free. The flour has superior nutritional value when compared to other grain-based flours, being rich in protein, fibre, magnesium, manganese and iron – it also makes great pancakes. These are similar to oatcakes in texture, and are flavoured with nori flakes and sesame seeds.

70 g/2½ oz. white sesame seeds
100 g/3½ oz. buckwheat flour
1 tablespoon chia seeds
1 teaspoon sea salt
1 tablespoon dried nori flakes
15 g/½ oz. black sesame seeds
1 tablespoon cold-pressed
   rapeseed oil
50 ml/3½ tablespoons water
freshly ground black pepper,
   to taste

*baking sheet, lined with baking
   parchment*

MAKES 12

Preheat the oven to 190°C (375°F) Gas 5.

Put the white sesame seeds in a mini food processor and process until they start to break down, about 2 minutes. Spoon them into a bowl and add the buckwheat flour, chia seeds, salt, nori flakes and black sesame seeds. Season with pepper and stir until combined, before adding the oil and water. Stir well with a fork and then form the mixture into a ball of dough with your hands.

Form the dough into a flattened round and place between two sheets of baking parchment. Using a rolling pin, roll the dough into a thin round, about 3 mm/⅛ inch thick and about 30 cm/12 inches in diameter. Mark the dough into 12 wedges with the pointed-end of a knife and prick the widest end of each with a fork. Place on the lined baking sheet and bake for 20–25 minutes until light golden and firm.

Using the marked lines, cut into 12 wedges and remove the buckwheat cakes from the baking sheet, using the baking parchment to help you. Leave to cool on a wire rack and then separate into individual cakes. Store in an airtight container for 3–5 days.

GRAIN-FREE 'CHEESY' PUMPKIN CRACKERS

Nutritional yeast flakes don't sound particularly appetizing, but they are nutritionally abundant and, despite being dairy-free, have a pleasant distinctly cheesy flavour that makes a useful addition to a vegan diet. The flakes are rich in both protein and B vitamins, which help with energy production.

90 g/3¼ oz. pumpkin seeds
2 large garlic cloves, skins peeled
10 g/¼ oz. poppy seeds or
    flaxseeds/linseeds
½ teaspoon sea salt
15 g/½ oz. nutritional yeast flakes
1½ teaspoons caraway seeds
1 tablespoon extra-virgin olive oil
50 ml/3½ tablespoons water
freshly ground black pepper,
    to taste

*baking sheet, lined with baking
    parchment*

MAKES 16

Preheat the oven to 190°C (375°F) Gas 5.

Put the pumpkin seeds and garlic in a food processor and process to a coarse paste. Add the rest of the ingredients, season with pepper and blend until the mixture starts to come together in a ball of dough.

Form the dough into a flattened rectangle and place between two sheets of baking parchment. Using a rolling pin, roll the dough into a square, about 3 mm/⅛ inch thick and mark the dough into 16 5-cm/2-inch squares with the pointed-end of a knife. Place on the lined baking sheet and bake for about 20–25 minutes until light golden and firm.

Using the marked lines, cut into 16 squares and remove from the baking sheet, using the baking parchment to help you. Leave to cool on a wire rack and then separate into individual crackers. Store in an airtight container for 3–5 days.

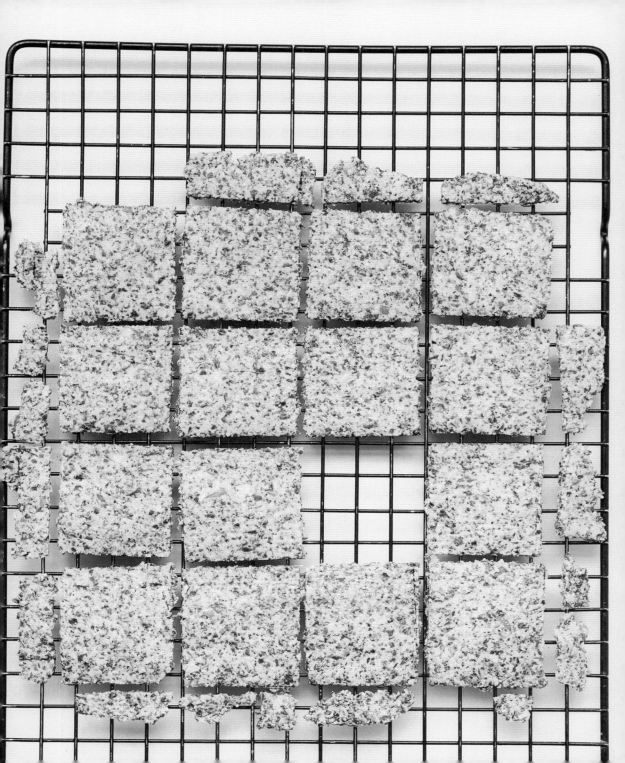

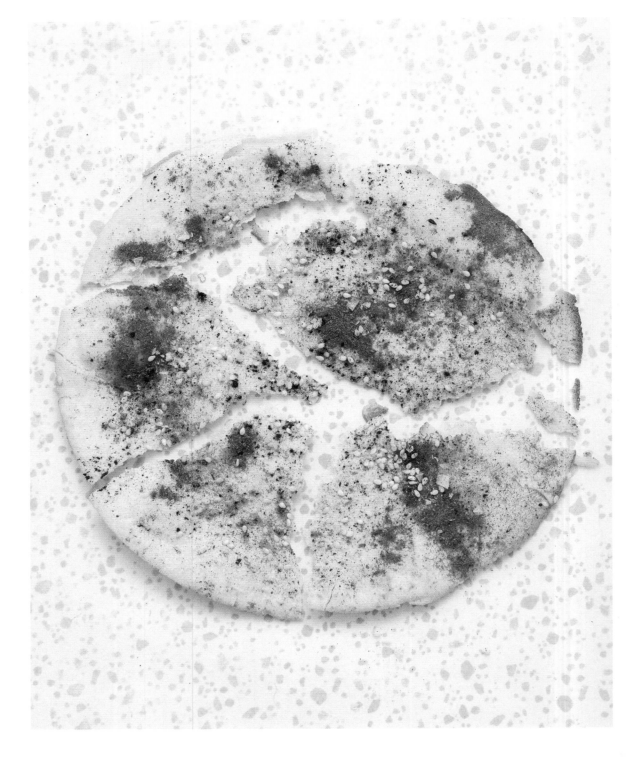

CAJUN TORTILLA CHIPS

Super-easy corn chips without the usual additives and flavourings, which are often found in shop-bought versions. They are flavoured with a homemade Cajun spice mix (you could use ready-made), as well as a sprinkling of spirulina and sesame seeds. You'll have leftovers of the Cajun spice mix, but it keeps well in a lidded jar for a couple of months or so.

4 corn tortillas
½ teaspoon spirulina powder
   (optional)
1 teaspoon sesame seeds
sea salt, to taste
extra-virgin olive oil, for brushing

CAJUN SPICE MIX
1 teaspoon dried oregano
1 tablespoon paprika
2 teaspoons ground turmeric
½ teaspoon chilli/chili powder
2 teaspoons ground cumin
1 teaspoon garlic granules/powder

SERVES 4

Preheat the oven to 180°C (350°F) Gas 4.

Mix together all the ingredients for the Cajun spice mix.

Place the tortillas directly on the shelves in the oven, spacing them apart so they don't touch each other. Bake for about 8 minutes, turning once, until crisp and golden in places. Remove from the oven and place on a wire rack.

Brush one side of each tortilla with oil and sprinkle over ¼ teaspoon of the Cajun spice mix, as well as the spirulina, if using, and some sesame seeds. Cut into wedges, then leave to cool and crisp up. They will keep in an airtight container for up to 2 days.

CAULI 'CHEESE' BITES

In addition to its wonderful colour, turmeric is a potent anti-inflammatory and antioxidant. The spice is more readily absorbed by the body when it's combined with fat, and its effectiveness is activated by piperine found in black pepper, both of which are used to make this simple snack.

5 teaspoons olive oil
1 teaspoon ground turmeric
250 g/9 oz. cauliflower florets
sea salt and freshly ground
   black pepper

VEGAN 'PARMESAN'
50 g/1¾ oz. pecan nuts
3 tablespoons nutritional yeast
   flakes

baking sheet, lined with baking
   parchment

MAKES 250 G/9 OZ.

Preheat the oven to 190°C (375°F) Gas 5.

Mix together the olive oil and turmeric, and season with salt and pepper.

Put the cauliflower in a bowl, pour over the turmeric mixture and turn until the florets are coated all over. Tip them onto the prepared baking sheet, spread out evenly and roast for 25–30 minutes, turning once, until tender and starting to colour.

While the cauli is roasting, make the vegan 'Parmesan'. Blitz the pecans and nutritional yeast flakes in a coffee or spice grinder to a coarse powder.

Spoon 2 tablespoons of the vegan 'Parmesan' over the roasted cauli and turn until evenly coated. (Any leftovers will keep in the fridge in an airtight container for up to 2 weeks.) The bites are best eaten warm but can be cooled and kept, covered, in the fridge for up to 2 days.

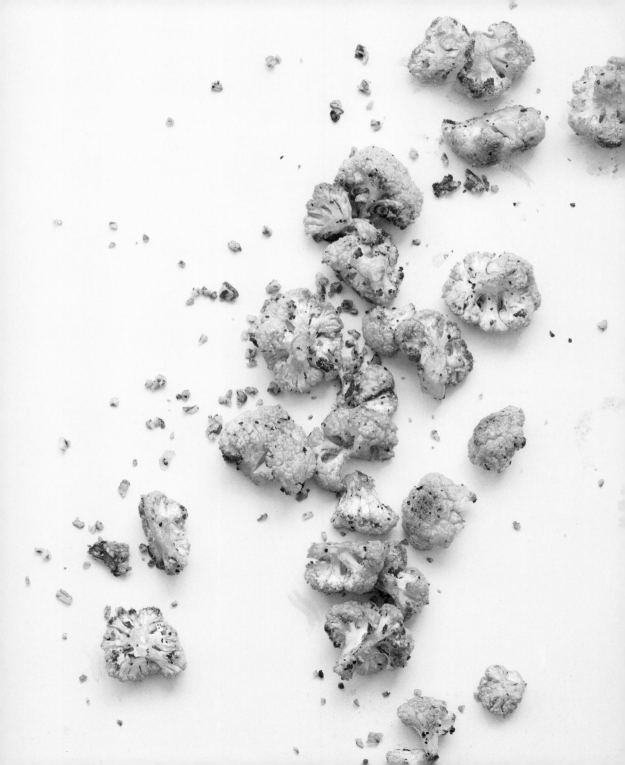

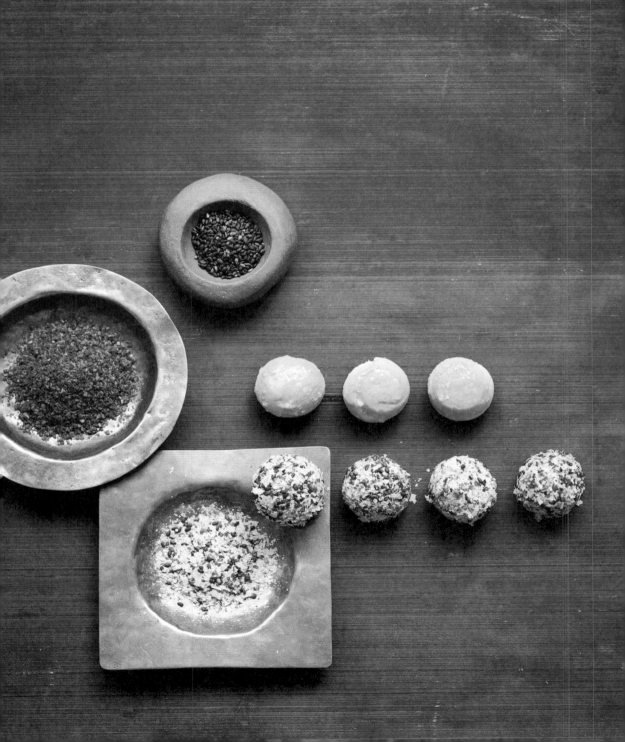

SAVOURY AVOCADO BITES

If you're looking for a quick and healthy savoury nibble, then these avocado bites tick all the right boxes. The balls are coated in a mixture of nutritional yeast flakes, black sesame seeds and red pepper flakes, and provide a good source of protein and beneficial fats, as well as a good range of vitamins and minerals. For the best flavour, eat soon after making, on their own or dunked into your favourite dip.

6 tablespoons nutritional yeast flakes
2 tablespoons black sesame seeds
1 teaspoon sweet red (bell) pepper flakes
large pinch of sea salt
freshly squeezed juice of 1 lemon
1 ripe avocado, cut in half and stone/pit removed

MAKES 6

Put the nutritional yeast flakes in a bowl, crushing any large flakes with the back of a fork. Stir in the sesame seeds, sweet red (bell) pepper flakes and salt.

Squeeze the lemon juice into a small bowl.

Using a melon baller or teaspoon, scoop the avocado flesh into 6 large, marble-sized balls, pressing them into a smooth round if needed.

Dunk each ball into the lemon juice as you go to prevent the avocado discolouring, and then dip into the nutritional yeast flake mixture until coated all over. Eat them straightaway or store, covered, in the fridge for up to 2 hours.

CORN CAKES WITH OLIVES & CHILLI/CHILE

Made from gram flour, this high-protein, gluten-free snack is a popular street food in Italy and southern France. Also known as socca, this version of the popular pancake is baked and cut into squares. It unconventionally contains egg, which gives a lighter texture than usual, and turmeric for a golden glow. It's topped with olives, cherry tomatoes, red onion and herbs, but feel free to add your own favourite toppings. It's also delicious served as a light meal with tzatziki or a zingy salsa on the side.

175 g/6 oz. gram flour
½ teaspoon sea salt
1 teaspoon ground turmeric
1 egg, lightly beaten
4 tablespoons olive oil
**1 red onion, thinly sliced into
rounds**
**1 red chilli/chile, deseeded and
thinly sliced**
**55 g/2 oz. pitted black olives,
halved**
10 cherry tomatoes, halved
**1 heaped tablespoon chopped
rosemary leaves**
**freshly ground black pepper,
to taste**

**30 x 25-cm/12 x 10-inch shallow
baking pan**

MAKES 15

Mix together the gram flour, salt and turmeric in a mixing bowl. Season with black pepper. Make a well in the centre and pour in 425 ml/scant 1¾ cups lukewarm water. Add the egg and half of the olive oil. With a balloon whisk, mix together the wet ingredients, then gradually draw in the flour mixture to make a smooth batter. Cover and leave to rest for 2 hours (or overnight in the fridge).

Preheat the oven to 220°C (425°F) Gas 7. Heat the remaining olive oil in the shallow baking pan for 5 minutes until very hot. Carefully remove from the oven and pour the batter into the pan.

Scatter the red onion, chilli/chile, olives, tomatoes and rosemary over the top. Bake for 15–20 minutes until set and golden. Leave to sit for a couple of minutes before cutting into 15 pieces, then remove and serve warm or cold. These will keep in the fridge in an airtight container for up to 3 days.

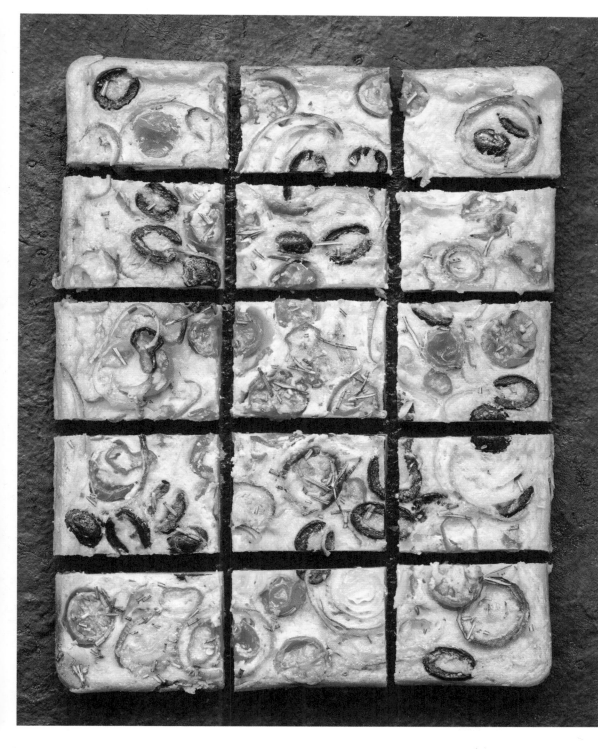

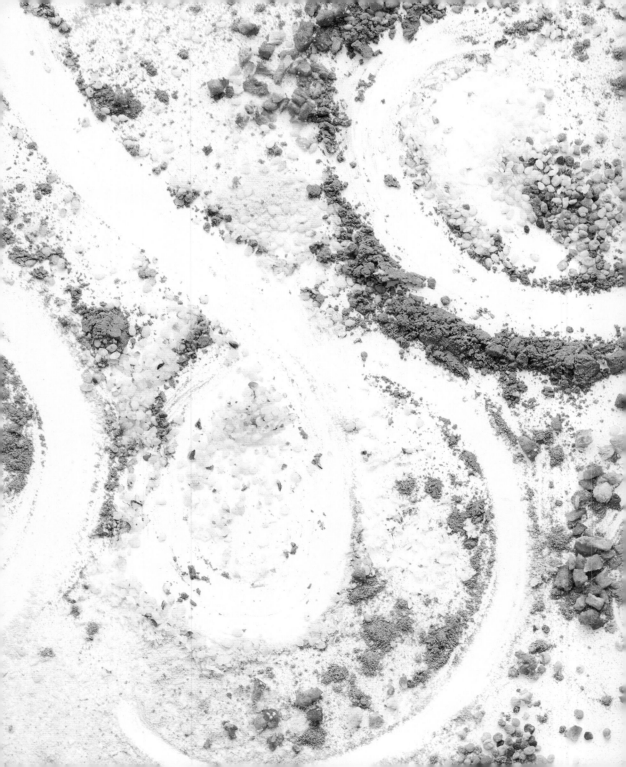

5

SUPERFOOD
TREATS

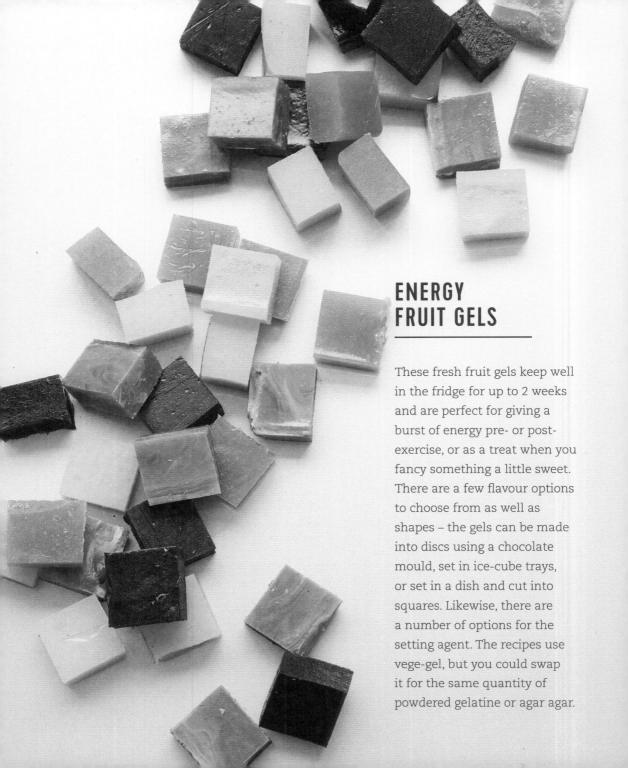

ENERGY
FRUIT GELS

These fresh fruit gels keep well
in the fridge for up to 2 weeks
and are perfect for giving a
burst of energy pre- or post-
exercise, or as a treat when you
fancy something a little sweet.
There are a few flavour options
to choose from as well as
shapes – the gels can be made
into discs using a chocolate
mould, set in ice-cube trays,
or set in a dish and cut into
squares. Likewise, there are
a number of options for the
setting agent. The recipes use
vege-gel, but you could swap
it for the same quantity of
powdered gelatine or agar agar.

NECTARINE & ROOIBOS GELS

South African rooibos tea comes with an impressive list of health benefits and is a potent anti-inflammatory and antiviral. Partnered perfectly with nectarines, this luscious fruit is brimming with immune-boosting vitamin C.

2 ripe nectarines
1 tablespoon powdered vege-gel
5 tablespoons cold rooibos tea
1–2 tablespoons good-quality
honey, to taste
bee pollen, for sprinkling
(optional)

mould, ice-cube tray or clingfilm-/
plastic wrap-lined shallow dish

MAKES ABOUT 14, DEPENDING ON THE SIZE OF THE MOULD

Place the nectarines in a heatproof bowl, pour over enough just-boiled water to cover, then leave for 1 minute. Scoop out the nectarines using a slotted spoon. When cool enough to handle, peel away the skins. Cut the fruit away from the central stones/pits and place in a blender. Blend to a smooth purée – you need about 125 ml/½ cup.

Pour the purée into a small saucepan and stir in the vege-gel until dissolved. Add the rooibos tea and 1 tablespoon of honey and heat gently, stirring, until the mixture almost reaches the boil and starts to thicken. Remove from the heat, taste and add an extra tablespoon of honey, if needed.

Place a mould, ice-cube tray or clingfilm-/plastic wrap-lined shallow dish on a work surface, then pour in the jelly mixture. Sprinkle over a few grains of bee pollen, if using, and place in the fridge to set. Pop the gels out of their mould or cut into 2-cm/¾-inch squares. Store in an airtight container in the fridge for up to 2 weeks.

RASPBERRY
KEFIR GELS

Kefir tastes like a slightly fizzy fermented yogurt. If that isn't selling it, then its amazing list of healthy properties might. It's a good source of protein, vitamin B12, calcium, magnesium, folate and probiotics, which support the digestive system and restore balance.

150 g/5½ oz. raspberries
1–2 tablespoons good-quality
honey, to taste
2 tablespoons thick kefir or live
yogurt
1 tablespoon powdered vege-gel

mould, ice-cube tray or clingfilm-/
plastic wrap-lined shallow dish

MAKES ABOUT 12, DEPENDING ON THE SIZE OF THE MOULD

Put the raspberries in a blender and blend to a smooth purée; you can pass the purée through a sieve/strainer to remove the seeds, if you like.

Pour the purée into a small saucepan and stir in the vege-gel until dissolved. Add 1 tablespoon of honey and heat gently, stirring, until the mixture almost reaches the boil and starts to thicken. Remove from the heat and stir in the kefir or yogurt, then taste and add another tablespoon of honey, if needed.

Place a mould, ice-cube tray or clingfilm-/plastic wrap-lined shallow dish on a work surface, then pour in the jelly mixture. Place in the fridge to set. Pop the gels out of their mould or cut into 2-cm/¾-inch squares. Store in an airtight container in the fridge for up to 2 weeks.

MANGO &
MACA GELS

The golden-hued mango makes this a perfect treat, being rich in vitamins C and A, dietary fibre and minerals. Maca has a balancing affect on the hormones and can aid endurance.

175 g/6 oz. prepared ripe mango, chopped
1 tablespoon powdered vege-gel
1–2 tablespoons good-quality honey, to taste
1 teaspoon maca powder

mould, ice-cube tray or clingfilm-/plastic
wrap-lined shallow dish

MAKES ABOUT 12, DEPENDING ON THE SIZE OF THE MOULD

Put the mango in a blender and blend to a smooth purée.

Pour the purée into a small saucepan and stir in the vege-gel until dissolved. Add 1 tablespoon of honey and heat gently, stirring, until the mixture almost reaches the boil and starts to thicken. Remove from the heat and stir in the maca, then taste and add another tablespoon of honey, if needed.

Place a mould, ice-cube tray or clingfilm-/plastic wrap-lined shallow dish on a work surface, then pour in the jelly mixture. Place in the fridge to set. Pop the gels out of their mould or cut into 2-cm/¾-inch squares. Store in an airtight container in the fridge for up to 2 weeks.

BLACK CHERRY
& ACAI GELS

Rich in antioxidants, including anthocyanins, these deep purple-coloured gels have anti-inflammatory and anti-ageing properties, and benefit overall health.

175 g/6 oz. frozen pitted black cherries,
defrosted
1 tablespoon powdered vege-gel
1–2 tablespoons good-quality honey, to taste
1 teaspoon acai powder

mould, ice-cube tray or clingfilm-/plastic
wrap-lined shallow dish

MAKES ABOUT 12, DEPENDING ON THE SIZE OF THE MOULD

Put the black cherries in a blender and blend to a smooth purée.

Pour the purée into a small saucepan and stir in the vege-gel until dissolved. Add 1 tablespoon of honey and heat gently, stirring, until the mixture almost reaches the boil and starts to thicken. Remove the pan from the heat and stir in the acai, then taste and add another tablespoon of honey, if needed.

Place a mould, ice-cube tray or clingfilm-/plastic wrap-lined shallow dish on a work surface, then pour in the jelly mixture. Place in the fridge to set. Pop the gels out of their mould or cut into 2-cm/¾-inch squares. Store in an airtight container in the fridge for up to 2 weeks.

FRUIT 'N' NUT CHOCOLATES

Make sure you choose a good-quality dark/bittersweet chocolate with a high percentage of cocoa solids to make these. The coconut oil lends a creaminess to the chocolate and while the acai is barely detectable taste-wise, it provides a range of nutrients, particularly antioxidants. As an added bonus, the top of each chocolate is decorated with good-for-you treats.

100 g/3½ oz. dark/bittersweet chocolate, about 85% cocoa solids, broken into squares
1 teaspoon coconut oil
1 tablespoon acai powder

TO DECORATE, CHOOSE FROM
bee pollen
goji berries
cacao nibs
toasted hazelnuts, roughly chopped

flexible chocolate mould, or baking sheet, lined with baking parchment

MAKES ABOUT 10, DEPENDING ON THE SIZE OF THE MOULD

Place the squares of chocolate and coconut oil in a heatproof bowl over a pan of gently simmering water, making sure the bottom of the bowl does not touch the water. Heat gently until the chocolate melts, stirring once or twice. Carefully remove the bowl from the heat and leave to stand for 3 minutes, then stir in the acai.

Pour or spoon the melted chocolate mixture into the flexible chocolate mould or spoon rounds onto the lined baking sheet.

Decorate with a sprinkling of bee pollen, goji berries, cacao nibs and/or toasted hazelnuts. Chill in the fridge until set, then transfer to an airtight container and keep in the fridge for up to 1 week.

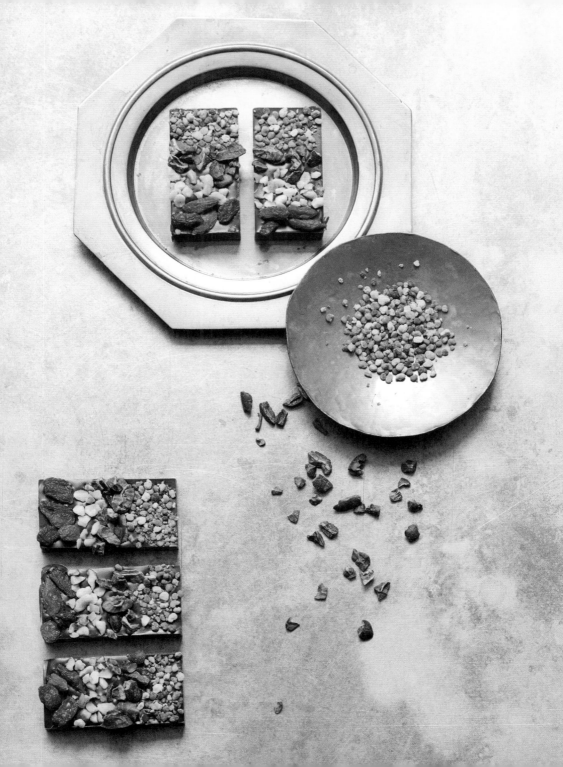

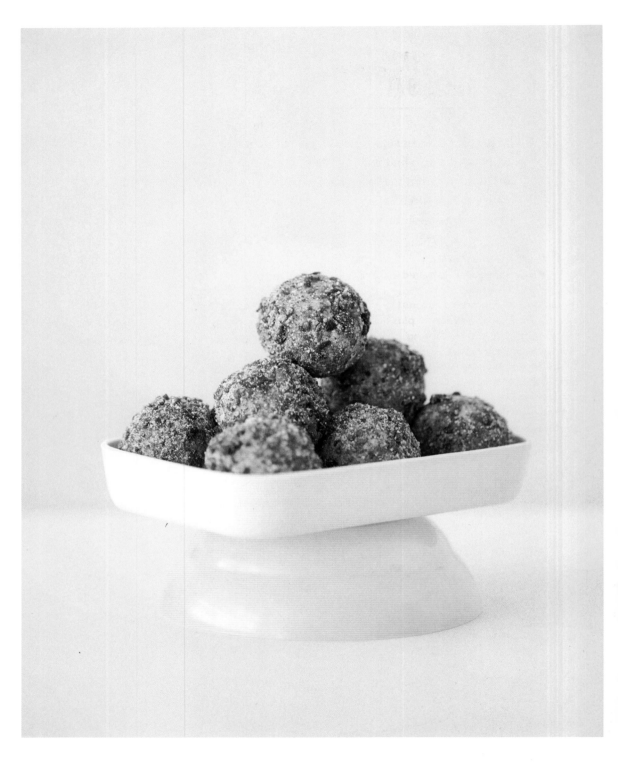

STRAWBERRIES & CREAM BALLS

Many of the larger supermarkets are now stocking raw cacao butter, and you can also find it in health food stores or online. The creamy aromatic fat from the cocoa bean is solid at room temperature and needs to be melted before use. A good source of antioxidants, it also provides magnesium, iron and vitamin E.

40 g/1½ oz. raw cacao butter
125 g/4½ oz. strawberries, hulled
50 g/1¾ oz. desiccated/dried
   unsweetened shredded coconut
100 g/3½ oz. ground almonds, plus
   extra 1 tablespoon for coating
1½ teaspoons pure vanilla extract
1 tablespoon good-quality honey
3 tablespoons freeze-dried
   strawberries, plus extra
   5 tablespoons for coating
1 tablespoon almond milk
   (optional)

MAKES 15

Gently melt the cacao butter in a small saucepan, then leave to cool slightly.

Purée the strawberries in a blender and then spoon them into a bowl. Stir in the coconut, ground almonds, vanilla, honey and freeze-dried strawberries. Stir in the almond milk if the mixture appears dry, bearing in mind it will firm up when chilled.

Mix together the remaining ground almonds and freeze-dried strawberries on a plate for coating.

With damp hands, shape the strawberry mixture into 15 walnut-sized balls, then roll each one in the dried strawberry mixture until coated all over. Chill for 30 minutes to firm up, then serve or store in the fridge in an airtight container for up to 1 week.

SALTED CARAMEL BANANA BITES

A cooling, protein-rich snack or indulgent after-dinner bite, the choice is yours, but there is no getting away from the fact that these are incredibly moreish.

125 g/4½ oz. peanut butter (crunchy or smooth)
3 tablespoons coconut oil
2 tablespoons maple syrup
2 bananas, peeled and roughly sliced
2 teaspoons maca powder (optional)
a handful of shelled unsalted pistachios, roughly chopped
sea salt flakes, for sprinkling

flexible chocolate mould or ice-cube tray

MAKES ABOUT 12, DEPENDING ON THE SIZE OF THE MOULD

Put the peanut butter, coconut oil, maple syrup, bananas and maca powder, if using, in a blender and blend until smooth and creamy.

Spoon the mixture into the flexible chocolate mould or ice-cube tray (the mixture should make about 12 in total), or another mould or container of your choice. Freeze for 1 hour until partially frozen, then remove and sprinkle the pistachios and a few sea salt flakes over the top. Return to the freezer until firm.

Once frozen, remove the banana bites from the mould or tray and store in a freezer bag or airtight container; they will keep for up to 1 month. For the best flavour, allow the banana bites to soften slightly before eating.

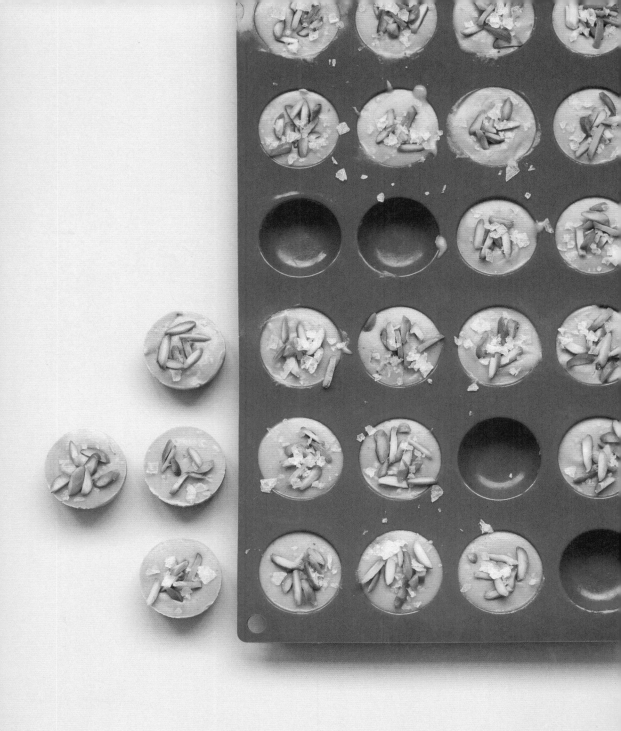

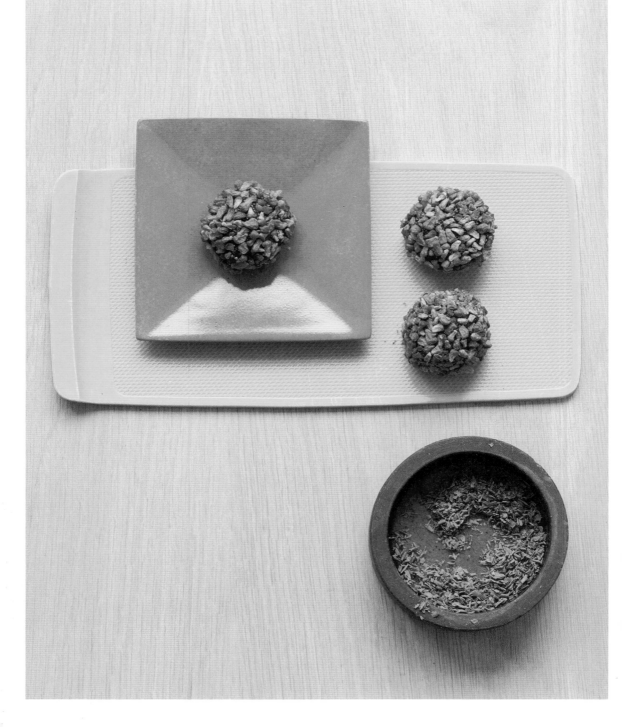

RAW CHOCOLATE & RASPBERRY TRUFFLES

These taste indulgently rich and special. Half the batch of truffles are coated in grated dark/bittersweet chocolate, while the other half are covered in freeze-dried raspberries. These are perfect for adding a burst of flavour, as well as colour, and can be found in the baking section of large supermarkets.

70 g/2½ oz. dark/bittersweet chocolate, about 70% cocoa solids
3 tablespoons coconut oil
4 tablespoons good-quality honey
100 g/3½ oz. raspberries
25 g/1 oz. raw cacao powder
1 tablespoon acai powder
6 tablespoons ground almonds
3 tablespoons freeze-dried raspberries, plus extra 4 tablespoons for coating

MAKES 22

Break 40 g/1½ oz. of the dark/bittersweet chocolate into even-sized pieces into a heatproof bowl. Add the coconut oil and honey, and heat gently over a pan of simmering water (make sure the bottom of the bowl does not touch the water) until melted, giving the mixture an occasional stir. Leave to cool slightly.

Mash the fresh raspberries to a rough purée, then stir into the melted chocolate. Add the cacao powder, acai powder, ground almonds and freeze-dried raspberries. Mix together until combined, then place the bowl in the fridge for 1 hour or until the mixture sets.

Grate the remaining dark/bittersweet chocolate onto a plate and place the remaining freeze-dried raspberries for coating on a separate plate.

Using a teaspoon, scoop a large, marble-sized portion of the chocolate mixture into the damp palm of your hand, and shape it into a ball. Roll it in the grated chocolate to coat, then repeat to make 11 chocolate-coated truffles.

Shape the remaining mixture as before, but roll them into the freeze-dried raspberries until coated. Chill the truffles for 30 minutes to firm up before serving and store in the fridge in an airtight container for up to 1 week.

DATE CARAMELS

Squares of sticky, creamy, toffee-like loveliness… these caramels derive their sweetness solely from dates. They contain almond flour, which has a finer texture than ground almonds, but if you have difficulty finding it, do swap it for the latter.

250 g/9 oz. soft dried pitted dates
**50 g/1¾ oz. almond flour or
 ground almonds**
2 tablespoons almond butter
2 teaspoons pure vanilla extract
**2 teaspoons lacuma or maca
 powder**
**¾ teaspoon sea salt flakes, plus
 extra for sprinkling**

*brownie pan, lined with clingfilm/
 plastic wrap, leaving enough
 overhang to cover the top*

MAKES 24

Put the dates in a bowl, pour over enough hot water to cover and leave to soften for 30 minutes.

Drain the dates well, pressing out any surplus water, then roughly chop. Place the dates in a food processor with the almond flour (or ground almonds), almond butter, vanilla, lacuma (or maca) powder and salt. Process until it forms a thick, smooth paste, occasionally scraping down the mixture from the sides, when needed.

Spoon the date mixture into the lined brownie pan and smooth with the back of a dampened spoon into an even layer, about 1 cm/½ inch thick. Fold the overhanging clingfilm/plastic wrap over the top.

Freeze for an hour or until firm, then lift out of the pan using the clingfilm/plastic wrap to help, cut into 24 2-cm/¾-inch squares and sprinkle the tops with a little extra sea salt. Store in the freezer in a freezer bag or airtight container for up to 1 month.

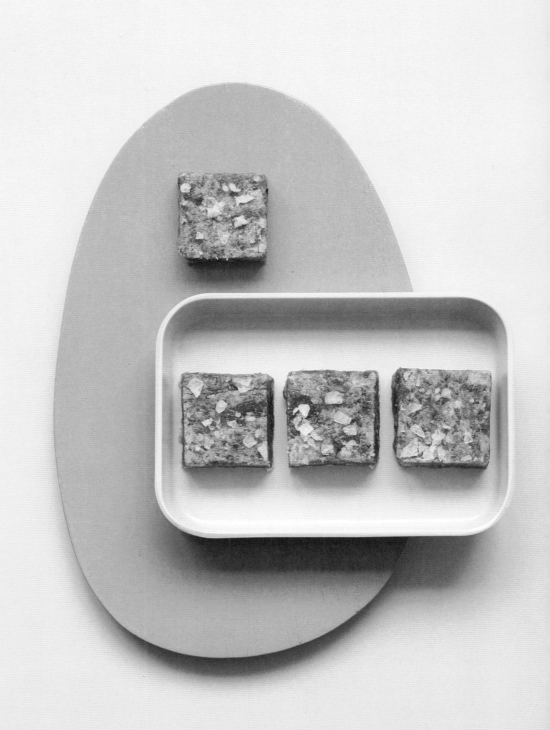

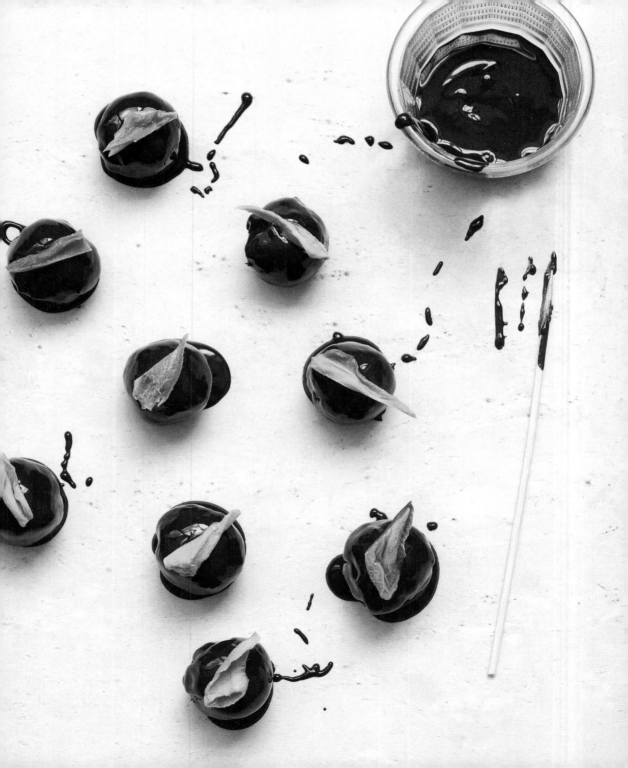